The 30-Minute

Sarah E. Moore

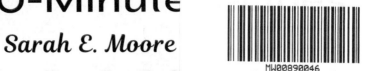

CELLULAR
HEALTH
COOKBOOK

Bring Dr Mercolas' Teaching To Your Table

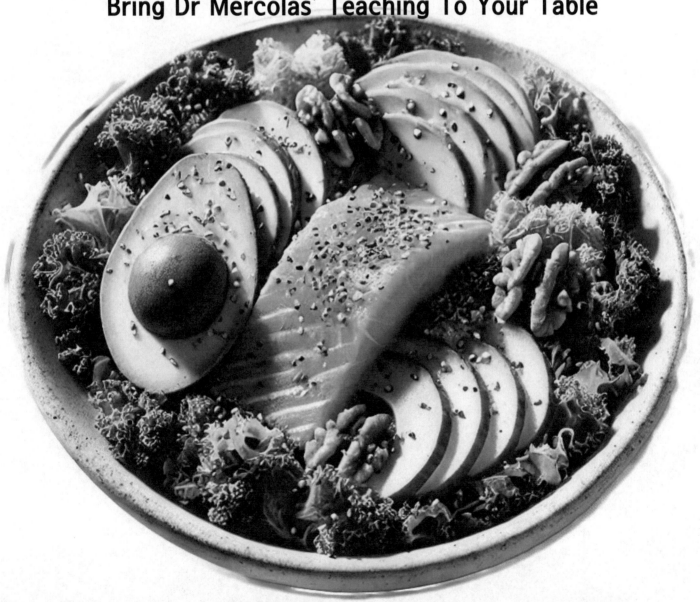

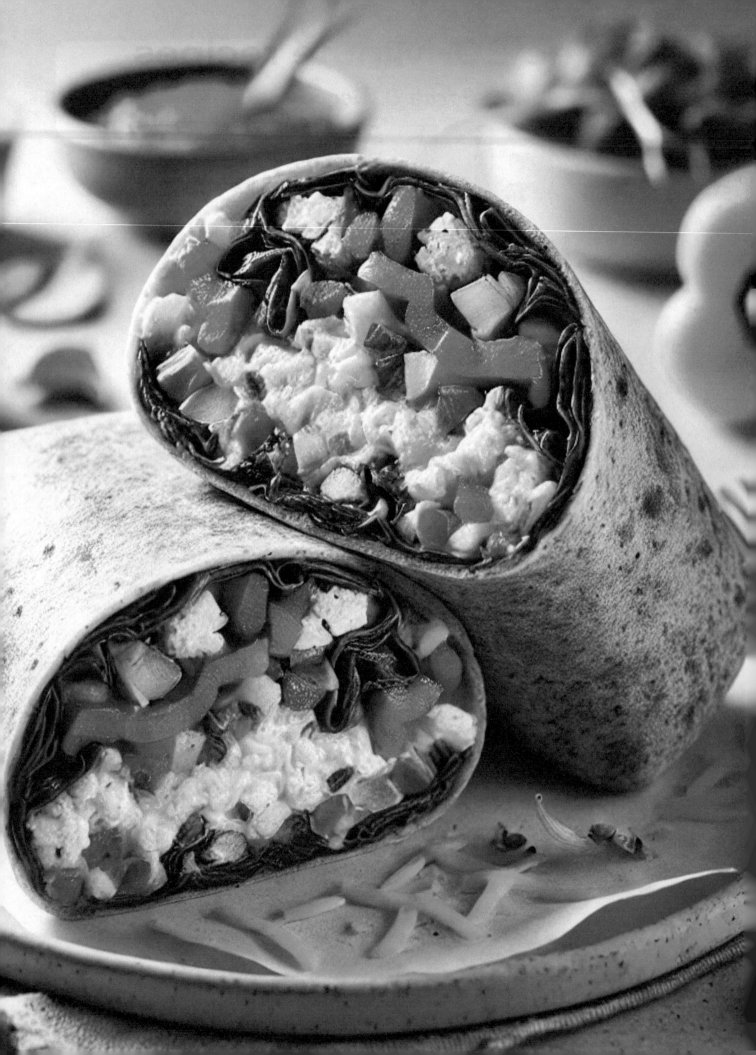

TABLE OF CONTENTS

TABLE OF CONTENTS

CHAPTER 1
CELL STRUCTURE AND FUNCTION
What is a Cell?

A cell is the basic unit of life. The study of cells, including their structure and the functions of their parts, is called Cell Biology. Robert Hooke was the first scientist to discover cells.

All living organisms are made of cells. They can either be made of one cell (unicellular) or many cells (multicellular). Mycoplasmas are the smallest known cells. Cells are the building blocks of life. They provide structure to the body and convert nutrients from food into energy.

Cells are complex, and each part of the cell has its own role. Just like bricks in a building, cells come in different shapes and sizes. Our body is made of cells of many shapes and sizes.

Cells are the smallest level of organization in any living thing. The number of cells varies from one organism to another. For example, humans have more cells than bacteria.

Inside cells, there are different parts called organelles that carry out specific tasks to keep the organism alive. Every organelle has its own structure. Cells also contain the genetic material that carries the organism's traits.

- Cells can sense and respond to their surroundings.
- Plant cells are adapted to protect themselves from external damage because they can't move. The cell wall helps with this.

Cell Wall
- The cell wall is a key part of plant cells. It's made of materials like cellulose, hemicellulose, and pectin.
- Only plant cells have a cell wall. It protects the cell's outer layer, including the plasma membrane and other components.
- The cell wall is a rigid layer that surrounds the cell membrane.
- It gives cells their shape, supports them, and protects them from damage.

Cytoplasm

- The cytoplasm is a thick, jelly-like substance inside the cell membrane.
- Most of the cell's chemical reactions happen in the cytoplasm.
- Organelles like the endoplasmic reticulum, vacuoles, mitochondria, and ribosomes float in the cytoplasm.
-

Nucleus
- The nucleus holds the cell's genetic material, called DNA.
- It controls the cell's activities, like when to grow, divide, or die.
- The nucleus is enclosed by the nuclear envelope, which separates the DNA from the rest of the cell.
- It protects the DNA and is a crucial part of the plant cell structure.

Functions of a Cell
A cell carries out many important functions that help an organism grow and develop. These include:

Provides Support and Structure
All organisms are made of cells, which give structure to the body. The cell wall and membrane provide support. For example, human skin is made of many cells. In plants, xylem cells give the plant its structure.

Facilitates Growth Through Mitosis
During mitosis, a cell divides to form new cells. This process helps the organism grow as the cells multiply.

Allows Transport of Substances
Cells take in nutrients to carry out chemical reactions. They also remove waste produced by these reactions. Small molecules like oxygen and carbon dioxide pass through the cell membrane by diffusion, a process called passive transport. Larger molecules require energy to move through the membrane, a process called active transport.

Energy Production
Cells need energy for chemical processes. Plants produce energy through photosynthesis, while animals get energy from respiration.

Aids in Reproduction

Cells help in reproduction through mitosis and meiosis. Mitosis is a type of asexual reproduction where a parent cell splits into two identical daughter cells. Meiosis, on the other hand, results in daughter cells that are genetically different from the parent.
Cells are known as the "structural and functional unit of life" because they provide the body with structure and carry out essential life processes.

CHAPTER 2
ENERGY PRODUCTION
What Do Mitochondria Do?

Mitochondria are involved in many processes, but their most well-known role is energy production. In fact, only about 3% of the genes that make up mitochondria are used for energy production. The rest are used for other tasks specific to the cell.

Here are some of the roles of mitochondria:

Producing Energy
ATP (adenosine triphosphate) is a complex molecule that powers metabolic processes. It is often called the "molecular currency" of energy. Most ATP is produced in the mitochondria through the citric acid cycle, also known as the Krebs cycle.

Energy production happens on the inner folds of the mitochondria, called cristae. Mitochondria turn the chemical energy from food into a form of energy the cell can use. This process is called oxidative phosphorylation.

During the Krebs cycle, a molecule called NADH is produced. NADH is then used by enzymes in the cristae to create ATP. Energy is stored in ATP's chemical bonds, and when these bonds break, energy is released for the cell to use.

Cell Death
Mitochondria also play a role in apoptosis, or programmed cell death. When cells get old or damaged, they are destroyed. Mitochondria decide which cells are removed by releasing cytochrome C, which activates caspase, an enzyme responsible for breaking down cells during apoptosis.
Certain diseases, like cancer, are linked to a breakdown in normal cell death (apoptosis), and because mitochondria help control this process, they may play a role in these diseases.

Storing Calcium

Calcium is essential for many cellular functions. For example, when calcium is released into a cell, it can trigger the release of neurotransmitters from nerve cells or hormones from endocrine cells. Calcium is also needed for muscle function, fertilization, and blood clotting, among other things.

Because calcium is so important, cells closely control its levels. Mitochondria help with this by absorbing calcium ions and holding them until the cell needs them. Calcium also helps with other functions like regulating cellular metabolism, steroid production, and hormone signaling.

Heat Production

When we are cold, our bodies can generate heat in different ways, including a process called non-shivering thermogenesis. Mitochondria generate heat through a process called proton leak. This is most common in brown fat, which is found in higher amounts in babies, as they are more sensitive to cold. As we age, the amount of brown fat decreases.

Mitochondria and Aging

In recent years, scientists have explored how mitochondrial dysfunction may be linked to aging. One popular theory is the mitochondrial free radical theory of aging. According to this theory, mitochondria produce reactive oxygen species (ROS) as a byproduct of energy production. These ROS can damage DNA, fats, and proteins in cells.

As mitochondria get damaged by ROS, they produce even more ROS, leading to more harm. This may contribute to aging, but not all scientists agree, and the exact role of mitochondria in aging is still unclear.

In Summary

Mitochondria are best known as the powerhouse of the cell, but they do much more than just produce energy. They are involved in calcium storage, heat production, and even the process of cell death, making them essential to many everyday cell functions.

CHAPTER 3
Oxidative Stress and Antioxidants
What is Oxidative Stress?

Oxidative stress occurs when your body's antioxidant levels are too low. Antioxidants and reactive oxygen species (ROS), or free radicals, need to stay balanced. When there are too many free radicals and not enough antioxidants, your body experiences oxidative stress. This can contribute to certain illnesses like diabetes.

Oxidative stress can cause cells and tissues to break down. However, in some cases, this imbalance may help fight conditions like cancer.

Why Are Antioxidants Important?
Antioxidants help protect your body from damage caused by free radicals. This protection is important for reducing the risk of diseases like heart disease, cancer, and other health problems.

Antioxidants are found naturally in vitamins like C and E, as well as in carotenoids, flavonoids, and tannins. You can get them from fruits, vegetables, nuts, seeds, whole grains, and spices. Antioxidants are also present in foods like cocoa, tea, and coffee.

Risk Factors for Oxidative Stress
When free radicals damage your cells, oxidative stress can have long-lasting effects. Some chronic diseases linked to oxidative stress include:
- Neurodegenerative diseases
- Diabetes
- High cholesterol (hypercholesterolemia)

Effects of Oxidative Stress on Health
Oxidative stress can have many negative effects on your health. Here are some conditions linked to oxidative stress:

Hypertension (High Blood Pressure):
Over 50 million Americans experience high blood pressure. Oxidative stress is believed to connect hypertension with atherosclerosis (the hardening of arteries). When certain enzymes that prevent oxidative stress are inactive, high blood pressure becomes more common.

Atherosclerosis:
This condition happens when free radicals damage blood vessels, causing inflammation. As a result, plaque builds up inside the arteries, increasing the risk of heart problems.

Heart Failure:
Oxidative stress can lead to heart failure by reducing antioxidant levels. This can cause harmful conditions like cardiac hypertrophy, cell death in the heart (apoptosis), and other heart issues that may worsen over time.

Stroke:
Studies show that oxidative stress can increase the risk of stroke by causing brain damage, known as ischemia-induced injury. With fewer antioxidants, the brain is more vulnerable to damage after a stroke.

Cardiovascular Disease (CVD):
Your risk of developing cardiovascular disease increases with oxidative stress. Factors like high blood sugar, obesity, smoking, poor diet, and stress can all raise the chances of CVD. Without enough antioxidants, cholesterol levels can rise, leading to clogged arteries and heart problems.

Cancer:
Oxidative stress can trigger changes in cells and molecules, leading to the development of cancer. The damage caused by ROS to DNA can encourage cancer cells to grow.

Neurological Diseases:
Oxidative stress has been linked to neurological diseases like Alzheimer's,

multiple sclerosis, and memory loss. Damage caused by free radicals can kill brain cells and speed up the progression of diseases like dementia. In Alzheimer's, for example, free radicals can create toxic proteins that damage the brain.

If you're concerned about oxidative stress, talk to your doctor. They can help you check your antioxidant levels and recommend whether you need antioxidant supplements.

CHAPTER 4
Cellular Aging (Senescence)
Understanding Cellular Aging

Cell aging, or senescence, happens as cells divide over time. This process is influenced by structures called telomeres and the aging process of cells.

Key Takeaways
- Telomeres shorten every time a cell divides, which limits the number of times a cell can replicate. This process is called replicative senescence.
- As we age, senescent cells (cells that stop dividing) build up and can contribute to age-related diseases and loss of tissue function.
- Telomere damage can happen even when their length is not reduced, contributing to the signs of cellular aging.

What Are Telomeres?

Telomeres are protective caps at the ends of chromosomes that help keep the genome stable. As cells replicate, these telomeres get shorter, eventually leading to a permanent stop in the cell cycle, known as replicative senescence. Senescent cells tend to build up in the body's tissues as we get older and are linked to age-related diseases. This means that the aging of cells may be part of why our tissues lose function with age.

This section will explore how telomeres can lead to cellular senescence and their role in responding to stress, regardless of their length.

Aging and Health

Key Facts About Aging
- Countries face major challenges in adjusting their healthcare systems for a rapidly aging population.
- By 2050, 80% of older adults will live in low- and middle-income countries.
- The aging population is increasing at a much faster pace than before.
- In 2020, there were more people over 60 than children under 5.
- By 2050, the global population over 60 years old will nearly double from 12% to 22%.

Overview of Global Aging Trends

Around the world, people are living longer. Today, many people can expect to live into their 60s and beyond. Every country is seeing a growth in both the number and proportion of older people.

By 2030, 1 in 6 people worldwide will be aged 60 or older. The global population over 60 will grow from 1 billion in 2020 to 1.4 billion. By 2050, the population over 60 will double to 2.1 billion, and the number of people over 80 will triple to 426 million.

This aging trend began in wealthier countries, but now low- and middle-income nations are seeing the greatest increase. By 2050, two-thirds of the global population over 60 will be in these countries.

What is Aging?

At the biological level, aging happens because of the build-up of damage in cells and molecules over time. This damage causes a gradual decline in physical and mental abilities, increased risk of diseases, and eventually death. The aging process isn't the same for everyone, and changes don't always occur at the same rate. Aging is also associated with life transitions, such as retirement, moving, and losing friends or partners.

Common Health Conditions Related to Aging

As people grow older, they tend to experience certain health conditions more often. These include:

- Hearing loss
- Cataracts and vision problems
- Back and neck pain
- Osteoarthritis
- Chronic obstructive pulmonary disease (COPD)
- Diabetes
- Depression
- Dementia

In addition to these, older people often deal with more complex conditions known as geriatric syndromes, which may include:

- Frailty
- Urinary incontinence
- Falls
- Delirium
- Pressure ulcers

Factors That Affect Healthy Aging

Living longer can provide many opportunities, such as pursuing new activities, education, or careers. Older people contribute a lot to their families and communities. However, enjoying these opportunities depends largely on health.

Health and Aging

Although people are living longer, evidence shows that many spend their extra years in poor health. If people can stay healthy as they age, they will be able to live similarly to younger individuals. But if their later years are marked by declines in physical and mental abilities, it can lead to negative outcomes for both individuals and society.

Most of the variation in health among older people is due to their physical and social environments, not genetics. Factors such as where people live, their socioeconomic status, and even their conditions before birth affect how they age.

The Role of Environment in Aging

Environments can impact health directly or indirectly by influencing behaviors and decisions. For example, staying physically active, eating a balanced diet, and avoiding smoking can all reduce the risk of diseases, maintain physical and mental capacity, and delay the need for care.

Supportive environments allow older people to stay active and do the things they value, even if they face physical challenges. Examples of supportive environments include safe, accessible public spaces, transportation, and walkable areas.

A good public health response to aging should not only address ways to reduce the effects of aging but also promote recovery, adaptation, and personal growth.

CHAPTER 5
THE SCIENCE OF CELLULAR REGENERATION: HOW OUR BODIES RENEW AND REPAIR THEMSELVES
Survival and Cellular Repair

In nature, survival often depends on an organism's ability to heal and repair itself. Since animals don't have access to medicine, the speed and effectiveness of their cellular repair is critical. Some animals have an impressive ability: cellular regeneration.

This process allows certain species to repair or even regrow damaged body parts. While humans have some regenerative abilities, such as skin repair, it is limited compared to animals like lizards, octopuses, and salamanders. Studying their regeneration helps us understand how we might improve our own.

The Basics of Cellular Regeneration

Cellular regeneration, or tissue repair, is a vital process for keeping organisms healthy. It involves replacing or repairing damaged or dying cells in the body. This process allows the body to heal injuries, recover from illnesses, and rejuvenate aging tissues.

Different cell types play key roles in regeneration. Stem cells are especially important because they can transform into various types of cells, replacing damaged ones. Other cells, like skin and muscle cells, help renew their specific tissues.

It's important to distinguish cellular regeneration from reproduction. Regeneration repairs damaged cells within an organism, while reproduction creates new organisms and cells.

In short, cellular regeneration keeps an individual alive, while reproduction ensures the survival of a species.

Factors Influencing Cellular Regeneration

Several factors influence how well our bodies can repair and regenerate cells. These factors affect our overall health and ability to heal.

A. Age and Regeneration

As we age, our body's ability to regenerate cells declines. This means slower healing and a higher risk of diseases. Understanding how age affects regeneration helps us develop ways to support it throughout life.

B. Nutrition, Exercise, and Lifestyle

Diet, exercise, and lifestyle choices greatly affect cellular repair. A diet rich in antioxidants, vitamins, and minerals supports regeneration, while poor habits, like a lack of exercise, can hinder it. Regular exercise increases blood flow and helps tissues heal, contributing to overall health.

C. Environmental and Genetic Factors

Environmental factors like exposure to toxins, pollution, and UV radiation can harm cells, making it harder for them to regenerate. Genetics also play a role in how well we can repair damaged cells. Understanding these factors helps us make better choices to boost regeneration.

Challenges and Limitations of Cellular Regeneration

A. Common Obstacles

One major obstacle is the natural decline in regenerative capacity as we age. Older cells don't replace damaged ones as efficiently, making it harder for the body to heal and function properly. In cases of severe injury or disease, the body's natural ability to repair itself may be insufficient, highlighting the need for advanced medical treatments like stem cell therapy.

B. Ethical Considerations in Stem Cell Research

Stem cell research holds great promise for cellular regeneration, but it also faces ethical challenges. The use of embryonic stem cells, for example, raises concerns about the destruction of embryos. Society must balance these concerns while exploring the potential of stem cells for healing.

C. Balancing Regeneration and Disease

There's a fine line between regeneration and uncontrolled cell growth, which can lead to diseases like cancer. If the mechanisms controlling cellular repair malfunction, it could trigger uncontrolled cell division. Understanding this balance is essential for safe regeneration.

Promoting Healthy Cellular Regeneration

Your body has an amazing ability to heal itself, and you can support this process through diet and lifestyle choices. Eating a balanced diet with nutrients like vitamins, minerals, and antioxidants helps your body repair damaged cells and tissues.

Exercise boosts blood circulation, delivering essential nutrients to cells and supporting regeneration. Rest is also crucial, as your body focuses on cellular repair while you sleep.

To optimize regeneration, avoid habits that harm your cells, such as smoking, excessive alcohol consumption, and chronic stress. Protect your skin from UV rays and pollution to reduce cellular damage. By making these changes, you can improve your body's ability to regenerate and maintain overall health.

The Role of Nutrition in Cellular Regeneration

A healthy diet plays a big role in cellular regeneration. Fruits and vegetables provide essential vitamins like C, A, and B vitamins. Whole grains offer minerals such as magnesium, zinc, and selenium. Lean proteins provide iron, zinc, and important B vitamins.

Proteins and Amino Acids

Proteins are essential for cell growth and repair. They are made up of amino acids, the building blocks of life. Amino acids help your body make new proteins, enzymes, and hormones necessary for cell function.

Eating enough high-quality proteins ensures your body has the amino acids it needs for cell repair. Foods like chicken, turkey, and fish provide essential amino acids, including lysine and tryptophan. Fish, such as salmon and tuna, are rich in omega-3 fatty acids, while dairy products like milk and yogurt are excellent sources of calcium and amino acids like leucine and valine.

Legumes (beans and lentils) offer a plant-based source of protein, while nuts like almonds and walnuts provide healthy fats and amino acids like arginine and tyrosine.

Incorporating these protein-rich foods into your diet supports your body's ability to repair tissues, produce enzymes, and maintain a strong immune system.

Improving Cellular Nutrition for Better Health

By improving your cellular nutrition, you can enhance your overall health. Consuming a variety of nutrient-dense foods, engaging in regular exercise, and taking care of your body can all contribute to better cellular regeneration and well-being.

Dietary Changes to Enhance Cellular Nutrition

Eating a nutrient-rich diet is essential for supporting your cells' function. This means focusing on whole foods that are full of vitamins, minerals, proteins, healthy fats, and carbohydrates. Limiting processed foods, sugary drinks, and unhealthy fats helps ensure your cells get the nutrients they need to stay healthy.

Lifestyle Modifications for Optimal Cellular Health

Along with diet, making lifestyle changes can also boost cellular health. Regular physical activity, managing stress, getting enough sleep, and avoiding smoking and too much alcohol all contribute to healthy cells and overall well-being.

The Long-term Effects of Poor Cellular Nutrition

Poor cellular nutrition over time can have serious effects on your health. It not only impacts how you feel day to day but also increases your risk of chronic diseases.

- Cardiovascular Disease: A lack of essential nutrients like antioxidants, omega-3 fatty acids, and fiber can lead to conditions like high blood pressure, atherosclerosis, and heart disease.
- Diabetes: Unhealthy eating habits, such as consuming too much sugar and processed foods, can cause insulin resistance and affect glucose metabolism, leading to type 2 diabetes.
- Cancer: Poor nutrition can weaken your body's defense against cancer. Nutrient deficiencies can prevent your body from repairing damaged cells and increase the risk of exposure to harmful substances.

- Accelerated Aging: Without enough antioxidants and nutrients to fight oxidative stress, aging speeds up, leading to wrinkles, age spots, and other signs of premature aging.

- Overall Quality of Life: Poor nutrition affects how your body and mind function. It can lead to low energy, mood swings, and a general feeling of unwellness, impacting relationships, work, and happiness.

- Weakened Immune System: A poor diet affects your immune system. Your immune cells need nutrients like vitamins A, C, and E to work properly. Without them, your body is more vulnerable to infections and illnesses.

CHAPTER 6
The Role of Exercise in Cellular Health

Exercise does more than change how you look; it also impacts your cells. Regular exercise supports healthy cell function and stimulates mitochondrial biogenesis (the creation of new mitochondria, the energy centers of your cells).

Cardio exercises, in particular, don't just benefit your heart—they also improve cellular health throughout your body. Here's how:

Cardio and Cellular Health

Cardiovascular exercise makes your heart pump faster and increases your heart rate, but it also has important benefits for your cells.

- Cardiac Cells: The cells in your heart muscle are highly specialized and don't regenerate often. Only about 1% of heart cells renew each year. However, studies show that cardiovascular exercise can promote heart cell growth.
-

In a 2018 study, researchers found that mice that ran regularly on a treadmill produced four times as many new heart cells as those that didn't exercise. This suggests that cardio exercise is crucial for supporting the health and regeneration of heart cells.

So, next time you want to improve your cellular health, consider adding some cardio to your routine—whether it's running, jogging, or swimming. Your heart cells will thank you!

Brain Cells and Exercise

Many people believe you can "train your brain" like a muscle, but while the brain has no muscle fibers, exercise does help improve brain function.

Exercise increases blood flow to the brain, providing more oxygen, which supports neuron growth and helps build new connections between brain cells. These new pathways are important for learning and memory, keeping the brain flexible.

Cardio exercises, in particular, benefit the brain by encouraging the growth of brain cells, much like strength training does for muscles. So, when you work out, you're not just improving your muscles—you're boosting your brain health too!

Immune Cells and Exercise

Exercise also helps your immune system by increasing the circulation of white blood cells (WBCs), which fight off germs. When you exercise, WBCs circulate more actively, helping to prevent illness. People who exercise regularly tend to catch fewer colds and other seasonal bugs.

However, it's important to exercise moderately. Intense workouts, like those of ultra-marathoners, can actually weaken the immune system, a condition known as overtraining syndrome. To find your ideal workout intensity, aim for 70% of your maximum heart rate. This will keep your immune system strong without overloading it.

Telomeres and Cellular Aging

Telomeres are the protective caps at the ends of your chromosomes, which contain your DNA. Over time, as cells replicate, telomeres shorten, which leads to aging and eventual cell death. Regular cardiovascular exercise can slow this shortening process, helping cells stay healthy longer.
Exercise increases the levels of telomerase, an enzyme that helps preserve telomeres. By boosting telomerase levels, exercise can help keep telomeres from shrinking too quickly, slowing down the aging process in your cells.

More Cellular Health Exercises—Strength Training

Cardio isn't the only exercise that benefits your cells. Strength training, like lifting weights or doing squats, also plays an important role in cellular health, especially for your muscle cells.

Muscle Cells and Strength Training

When you do strength training, tiny injuries occur in your muscle cells. This might sound bad, but these micro-injuries actually help your muscles grow stronger. Nearby satellite cells jump into action, fusing with the injured muscle cells and donating their mitochondria and nuclei to help with repair.

This process allows muscle cells to produce more energy and force, helping your muscles grow stronger over time. Without strength training, your muscles wouldn't benefit from this repair and growth.

Reap the Cellular Benefits of Exercise

When you exercise regularly, your body benefits in ways you can see, like improved strength and fitness. But below the surface, your cells are also thriving. Every workout—whether it's cardio or strength training—helps the trillions of cells in your body function better.

So next time you exercise, remember that you're helping not just your muscles and heart, but every single cell in your body!

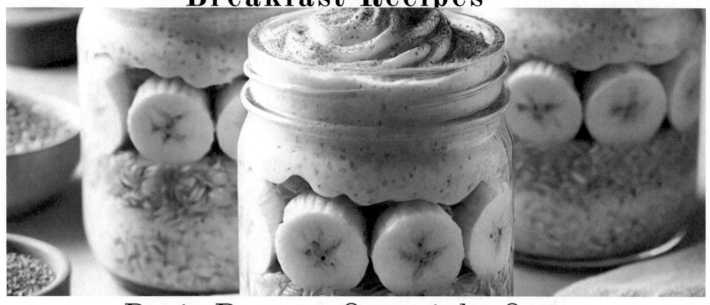

Basic Banana Overnight Oats

Directions

Ingredients

Prep Time: 10 minutes

Cook Time: 12 hours (overnight)

Total Time: 12 hours

Yield: 4 servings

Category: Breakfast

Method: No-cook

Ingredients:

- 2 cups old-fashioned rolled oats
- 4 cups oat milk (or any milk of your choice)
- 1 ripe banana (mashed)
- 2 tbsp chia seeds
- 2 tsp ground cinnamon
- Pinch of kosher sea salt

Prepare Jars:

1. Line up four mason jars or food storage containers. Divide the ingredients evenly between each jar. Add 1/2 cup oats, 1 cup milk, 1/4 banana, 1/2 tbsp chia seeds, 1/2 tsp cinnamon, and a pinch of salt into each jar. Stir everything well to combine.

Refrigerate:

1. Cover the jars with lids and refrigerate overnight or for up to two days. You can eat them as they are or add your favorite toppings before serving.

Notes:

1. Feel free to use any milk of your choice, like almond or cow's milk, depending on your preference.
2. The nutrition information is for the base recipe without toppings.

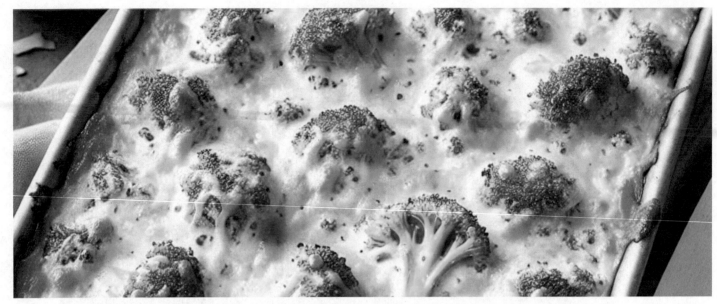

Easy Broccoli and Cheese Egg Bake

Ingredients

Prep Time: 10 minutes

Cook Time: 35 minutes

Total Time: 45 minutes

Servings: 12 servings

Calories: 129 kcal per serving

Ingredients:

- 12 eggs
- 1 cup milk (cow's milk or almond milk)
- 1 small onion (diced)
- 2 heaping cups broccoli florets (chopped)
- 1 ½ cups shredded cheese (Mexican blend or cheddar recommended)
- ¼ tsp salt (or more to taste)
- ¼ tsp ground black pepper (or more to taste)

Directions

Preheat Oven:

Set your oven to 400°F and lightly spray a 9x13 baking dish with oil.

Mix Ingredients:

In a large bowl, whisk together the eggs and milk. Stir in the chopped broccoli, onions, shredded cheese, salt, and pepper until well combined.

Bake:

Pour the mixture into the prepared baking dish and bake for about 25-30 minutes or until the eggs are cooked through. Let the dish stand for 5-10 minutes before serving.

Notes:

- You can prepare this dish a day in advance. Just cover it tightly with foil and refrigerate until ready to bake.

Store leftovers in an airtight container in the fridge and reheat in the microwave for 1-2 minutes.

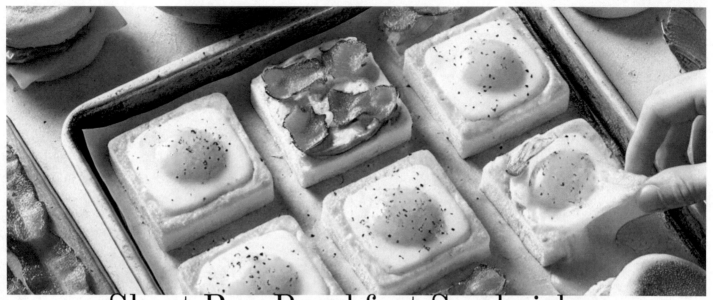

Sheet Pan Breakfast Sandwiches

Ingredients

Prep Time: 5 minutes

Cook Time: 15 minutes

Total Time: 30 minutes

Servings: 12 servings

Ingredients:

- 12 large eggs
- 1/2 cup whole milk
- 6 oz cheese (your choice)
- Nonstick spray
- Salt and pepper (to taste)
- Avocado
- English muffins
- Bacon (optional)

Directions

1. Preheat Oven:

 Preheat your oven to 375°F. Whisk the eggs and milk together until smooth.

2. Bake the Eggs:

 Spray a sheet pan with nonstick spray and pour the egg mixture onto the pan. Bake for 12 minutes. The eggs should be mostly cooked but still slightly liquid.

3. Add Cheese:

 Remove the pan from the oven, add the cheese, and return it to the oven for 3 more minutes to melt the cheese and finish cooking the eggs.

4. Prepare for Freezing:

 Once the eggs are completely cool, cut them into 12 squares. Wrap each square in plastic and freeze them. For long-term storage, wrap the squares in foil as well.

5. Reheat and Assemble:

 To reheat, remove the plastic and microwave the egg square for about a minute. Add the egg to a toasted English muffin along with avocado and bacon (if using) for a quick sandwich.

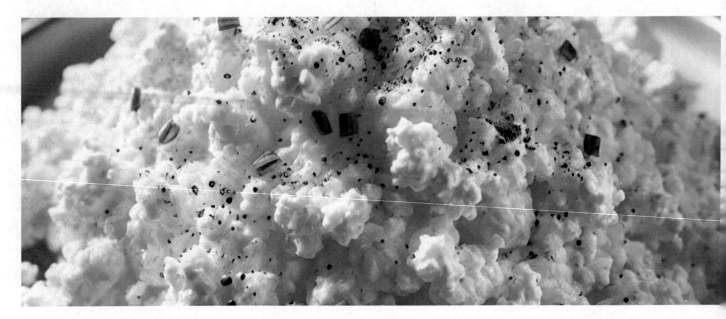

The Ultimate High Protein Scrambled Eggs

Ingredients

Prep Time: 5 minutes

Cook Time: 2 minutes

Total Time: 7 minutes

Ingredients:

- 4 large eggs
- 2/3 cup plain low-fat cottage cheese
- 1/4 tsp kosher salt
- 1/8 tsp freshly ground black pepper
- 1 tsp chopped fresh chives (optional)
- 1 tbsp extra-virgin olive oil

Directions

1.Mix Ingredients:
 In a bowl, whisk together the eggs, cottage cheese, salt, pepper, and chives (if using).

2.Cook Eggs:
 Heat a medium nonstick skillet over medium heat. Add the olive oil and pour in the egg mixture. Use a spatula to gently scrape the eggs toward the center as they cook. The eggs should be done in about 2 minutes.

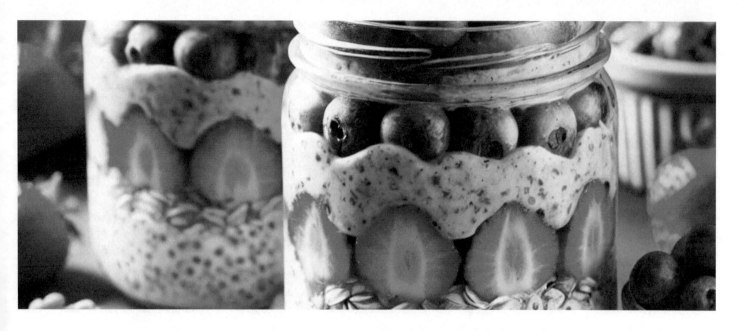

Berry and Chia Overnight Oats

Ingredients

Prep Time: 5 minutes

Total Time: 4 hours (or overnight)

Ingredients:

- 2/3 cup milk
- 1/3 cup plain nonfat Greek yogurt
- 1 cup old-fashioned oats
- 1 tbsp chia seeds
- 1/2 medium banana (mashed)
- 1 cup fresh blueberries
- 1 cup fresh sliced strawberries
- 1/4 cup chopped walnuts

Directions

1.Mix Base:

 In a bowl, combine the milk, yogurt, oats, chia seeds, and mashed banana. Stir well.

2.Divide and Chill:

 Divide the mixture into two jars or containers. Top with half the blueberries, strawberries, and walnuts. Refrigerate for at least 4 hours or overnight.

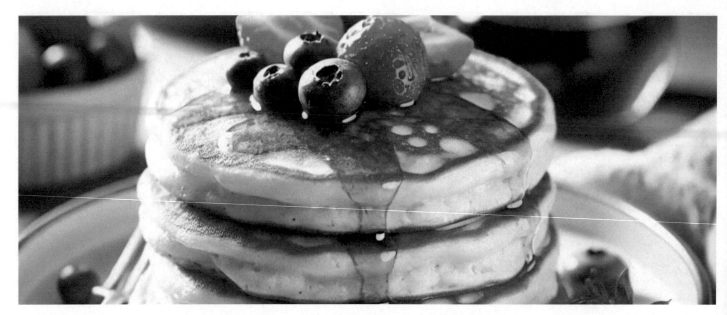

Light and Fluffy Cottage Cheese Pancakes

Ingredients

Prep Time: 5 minutes

Cook Time: 10 minutes

Total Time: 15 minutes

Ingredients:

- 1 cup old-fashioned rolled oats (gluten-free if desired)
- 1 cup plain low-fat cottage cheese
- 4 large eggs
- 2 tsp baking powder
- 1 tsp pure vanilla extract
- 1/4 tsp kosher salt
- 2 tbsp pure maple syrup
- 2 tbsp canola oil

Directions

1. Blend Ingredients:

Place all ingredients (except oil) in a blender or food processor and blend on high until smooth (about 30-60 seconds).

2. Cook Pancakes:

Heat a nonstick skillet over medium heat. Add a little oil and pour the batter to form small pancakes. Cook until bubbles form in the center (about 1 minute), flip, and cook until golden brown (about another minute). Serve with fresh fruit or toppings of your choice.

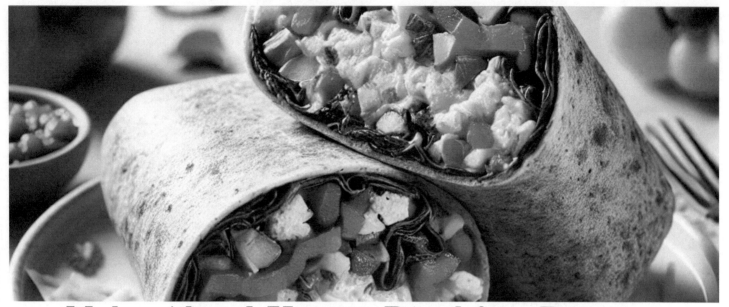

Make-Ahead Veggie Breakfast Burrito

Ingredients

Prep Time: 5 minutes

Cook Time: 10 minutes

Total Time: 15 minutes

Ingredients:

- 1 tbsp extra-virgin olive oil
- 1 red bell pepper (diced)
- 2 shallots (diced)
- 2 cloves garlic (minced)
- 2 cups baby spinach
- 12 large eggs
- 1 pinch kosher salt
- 1/4 tsp freshly ground black pepper
- 4 whole-wheat tortillas

1/2 cup shredded cheddar cheese

Directions

1. Cook Veggies:

Heat a medium skillet over medium heat. Add olive oil, then sauté the bell pepper, shallots, and garlic for 5–7 minutes until soft. Stir in the spinach and cook for 1–2 minutes until wilted.

2. Cook Eggs:

In a bowl, whisk the eggs with salt and pepper. Pour into the skillet with the veggies and cook over medium-low heat, stirring frequently until the eggs are set (about 3–5 minutes).

3. Assemble Burritos:

Divide the egg mixture evenly among the tortillas. Top each with 2 tablespoons of cheese. Fold the tortillas and roll them tightly.

4. Optional:

If you like crispy tortillas, cook the burritos in a clean skillet for 1–2 minutes on each side until lightly browned.

Tip: To make this a grab-and-go breakfast, let the burritos cool, wrap them in plastic wrap, and freeze. Defrost in the fridge overnight and reheat in the microwave for 1–2 minutes, or cook in a skillet for 2–3 minutes per side.

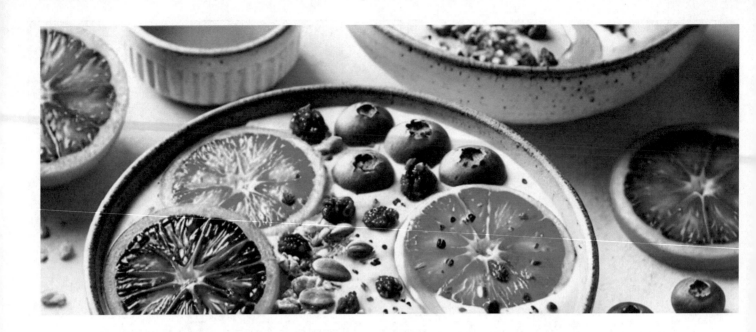

Winter Citrus Yogurt Bowl

Ingredients

Prep Time: 5 minutes

Total Time: 5 minutes

Ingredients:

- 2 cups plain nonfat Greek yogurt
- 1 blood orange (peeled and sliced)
- 1/4 cup granola
- 2 tbsp pepitas (or other nuts/seeds)
- 1/4 cup fresh blueberries
- 1 tbsp honey (optional)

Directions

1. Assemble:

Divide the yogurt into two bowls. Top each with half the orange slices, granola, pepitas, and blueberries. Drizzle with honey if desired.

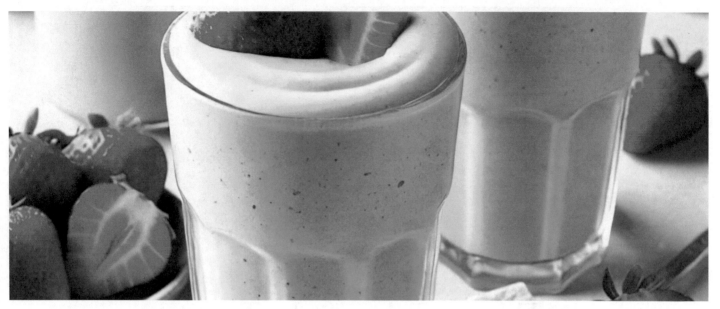

Strawberry Cream Smoothie

Ingredients

Prep Time: 5 minutes

Total Time: 5 minutes

Ingredients:

- 2 cups frozen strawberries
- 2 cups plain unsweetened soy milk
- 9 oz extra-firm silken tofu (drained)
- 2 tbsp sunflower seed butter (or peanut butter)
- 1 tsp pure vanilla extract
- Sliced strawberries (optional topping)

Directions

1.Blend:
 Add all ingredients to a blender and blend on high until completely smooth.
2.Serve:
 Divide between two glasses and top with sliced strawberries if using.

33

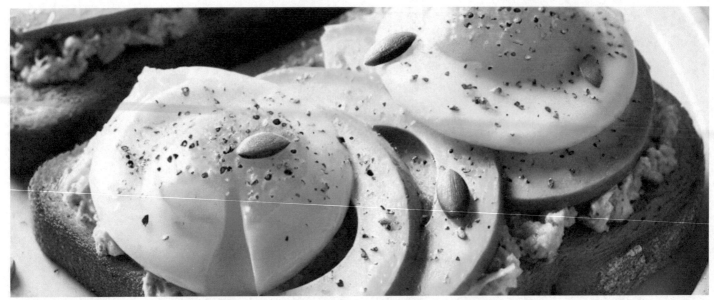

Egg and Avocado Toast

Ingredients

Prep Time: 3 minutes

Cook Time: 5 minutes

Total Time: 8 minutes

Ingredients:

- 1 slice whole-wheat bread
- 1 tsp mayonnaise (olive oil-based preferred)
- 1/4 avocado (sliced)
- 2 eggs (cooked to your liking)
- Pinch of kosher salt
- Pinch of freshly ground black pepper
- 1 tbsp pepitas (optional garnish)

Directions

1.Toast Bread:

 Toast the bread to your preferred crispness, then spread the mayonnaise evenly on top.

2.Assemble:

 Top with avocado slices and cooked eggs.

Sprinkle with salt, pepper, and pepitas (if using).

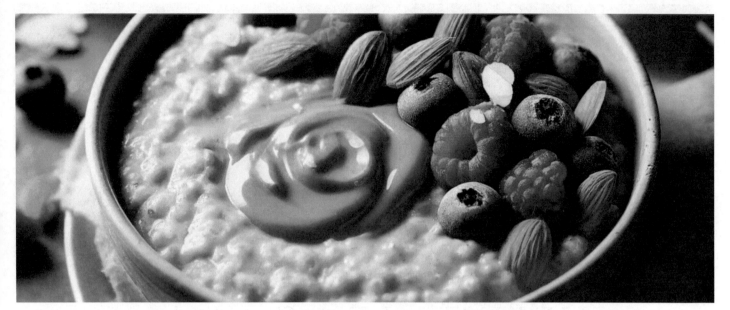

Almond Butter Oatmeal

Ingredients

Prep Time: 5 minutes

Cook Time: 25 minutes

Total Time: 30 minutes

Ingredients:

- 3 cups unsweetened vanilla soy milk (or almond milk)
- 1 cup dry steel-cut oats
- 3 tbsp smooth almond butter
- 1/4 tsp salt
- 2 cups fresh berries (of your choice)

Directions

1.Cook Oats:

 In a medium pot, bring the soy milk to a boil. Stir in the oats, return to a boil, then reduce heat to simmer. Cover and cook for 25–30 minutes, stirring occasionally until the liquid is absorbed.

2.Finish:

 Remove from heat and stir in almond butter and salt. Serve with fresh berries.

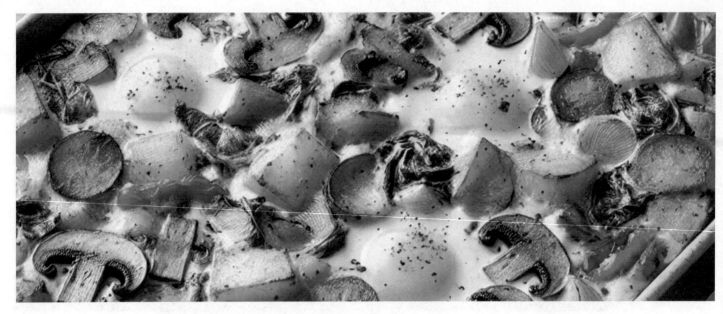

Make-Ahead Egg Casserole

Ingredients

Prep Time: 10 minutes

Cook Time: 50 minutes

Total Time: 1 hour

Ingredients:

- 12 large eggs
- 1/2 cup nonfat milk (or nondairy milk)
- 1 tsp kosher salt
- 1 tsp garlic powder
- 1/2 tsp freshly ground black pepper
- 2 tbsp extra-virgin olive oil
- 1 lb new potatoes (quartered)
- 1 small yellow onion (sliced)
- 1 cup sliced mushrooms
- 1 bell pepper (diced)
- 2 cups baby spinach

Directions

1.Prepare Eggs:

 In a large bowl, whisk together the eggs, milk, salt, garlic powder, and pepper. Set aside.

2.Cook Veggies:

 Heat a skillet over medium heat. Add olive oil, potatoes, and onion. Cook for 5–7 minutes until the onion is translucent. Add mushrooms and bell pepper, cooking for another 5 minutes.

3.Assemble Casserole:

 Spray a baking dish with cooking spray. Add the cooked veggies and top with spinach. Pour in the egg mixture. Refrigerate until ready to bake.

Bake:

 Preheat the oven to 350°F and bake for 40–50 minutes until the eggs are set.

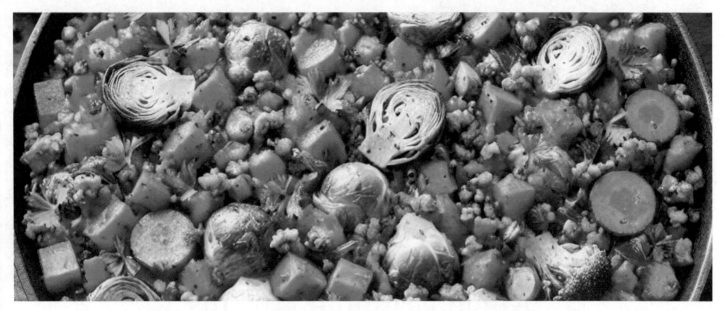

Sweet Potato Breakfast Hash

Ingredients

- 1 tbsp avocado oil
- 1 large sweet potato (peeled and diced)
- 2 carrots (sliced)
- 1/2 cup Brussels sprouts (quartered)
- 3-4 cloves garlic (minced)
- 1 tsp marjoram
- 1 tsp sea salt (plus more to taste)
- 1 lb ground turkey
- Fresh parsley (for topping)

Directions

1.Cook Veggies:
 Heat the avocado oil in a large pan over medium heat. Add the sweet potatoes and carrots, cooking for 10 minutes. Then add Brussels sprouts, garlic, marjoram, and salt. Cook for another 5 minutes.

2.Cook Turkey:
 Add the ground turkey to the pan and break it apart with a spatula. Cook for 5-7 minutes or until the turkey is fully cooked.

3.Serve:
 Top with fresh parsley and serve.

Note: Feel free to mix and match veggies and meat based on what you have on hand.

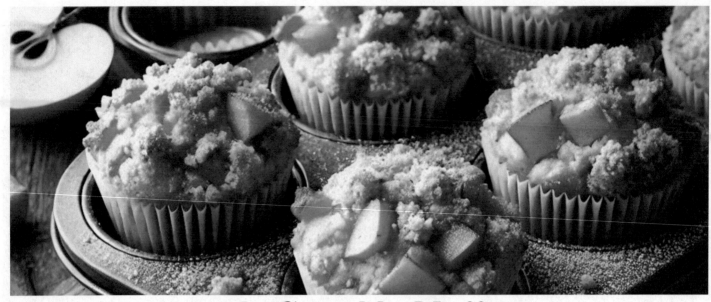

Apple Crumble Muffins

Ingredients

- 1 cup cassava flour
- 1/2 cup tigernut flour
- 1/2 cup arrowroot flour
- 2 tsp baking soda
- 1/2 tsp cream of tartar
- 2 tbsp gelatin
- 1 tsp cinnamon
- 1/2 cup applesauce
- 1/2 cup coconut oil
- 2 ripe bananas (chopped)
- 1/2 cup maple syrup
- 1/4 cup water or full-fat coconut milk
- 1 cup chopped apples
- Coconut sugar (for sprinkling)

Directions

1. Preheat Oven: Preheat the oven to 350°F.
2. Mix Dry Ingredients: In a large mixing bowl, combine the cassava flour, tigernut flour, arrowroot flour, baking soda, cream of tartar, gelatin, and cinnamon.
3. Mix Wet Ingredients: In a separate bowl, combine applesauce, coconut oil, bananas, maple syrup, and water or coconut milk. Blend until smooth if desired.
4. Combine Mixtures: Add the wet ingredients to the dry ingredients and mix until well combined.
5. Add Apples: Fold in the chopped apples.
6. Prepare Muffin Tin: Line a muffin pan with liners and spoon the batter into each, shaping as needed.
7. Bake: Sprinkle with coconut sugar and bake for 25 minutes for mini muffins or 35 minutes for regular-sized muffins.

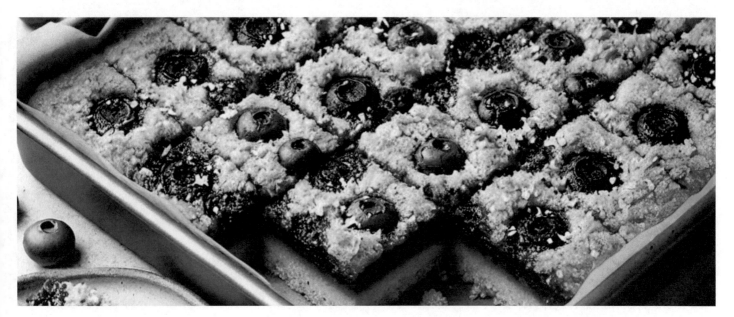

Blueberry AIP-Paleo Breakfast Bars

Ingredients

Crust:

- 1/2 cup coconut flour
- 1/4 cup arrowroot flour
- 1 tbsp gelatin
- 1 tbsp maple syrup
- 2 tbsp coconut oil (melted)
- 1/4 cup coconut milk
  (more if needed)

Filling:

- 4 tsp arrowroot flour
- 1/2 cup maple syrup
- 4 cups frozen wild
  blueberries
- 2 tsp vanilla extract

Topping:

- 1 cup coconut flour
- 1/4 cup coconut oil
- 2 tbsp coconut sugar

Directions

1.Preheat Oven: Preheat the oven to 350°F.

2.Prepare Crust: In a medium bowl, combine the crust ingredients. Press into an 8x8 baking pan lined with parchment paper. Bake for 5 minutes.

3.Prepare Filling: In another bowl, mix the filling ingredients.

4.Prepare Topping: Mix the topping ingredients in a small bowl.

5.Assemble: Add the filling over the baked crust, then sprinkle the topping over it.

6.Bake: Bake for 25-30 minutes. Let cool before cutting and serving.

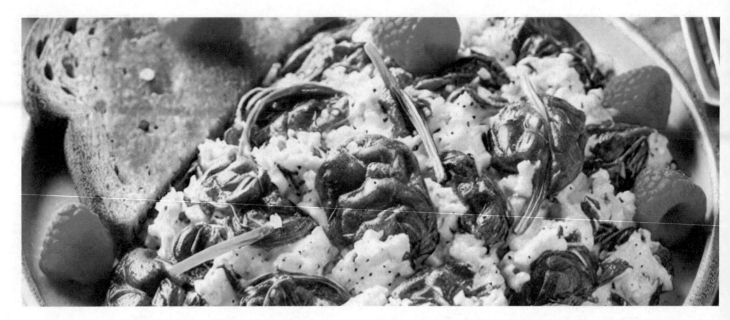

Spinach & Egg Scramble with Raspberries

Ingredients

- 1 tsp canola oil
- 1 1/2 cups baby spinach
- 2 large eggs (lightly beaten)
- Pinch of kosher salt
- Pinch of ground pepper
- 1 slice whole-grain bread (toasted)
- 1/2 cup fresh raspberries

Directions

1. Cook Spinach: Heat oil in a small skillet over medium-high heat. Add spinach and cook until wilted (1-2 minutes).
2. Cook Eggs: Wipe the skillet clean and scramble the eggs with salt and pepper over medium heat (1-2 minutes). Stir in the spinach.
3. Serve: Serve the scramble with toast and fresh raspberries.

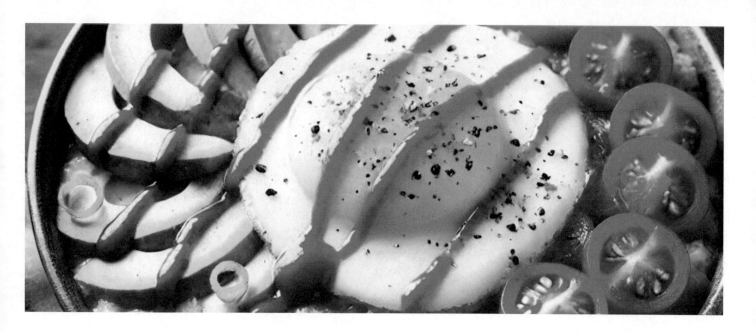

Sriracha, Egg & Avocado Overnight Oats

Ingredients

- 1/2 cup rolled oats
- 3/4 cup water
- 1 tbsp diced onion
- 1/4 avocado (sliced)
- 2 cherry tomatoes (chopped)
- 1 large egg (fried)
- 1 tsp Sriracha

Directions

1.Prepare Oats:
 Combine oats and water in a bowl or jar, cover, and refrigerate overnight.

2.Assemble:
In the morning, stir in the onion and heat the oats in the microwave in 30-second intervals. Top with avocado, tomatoes, fried egg, and Sriracha.

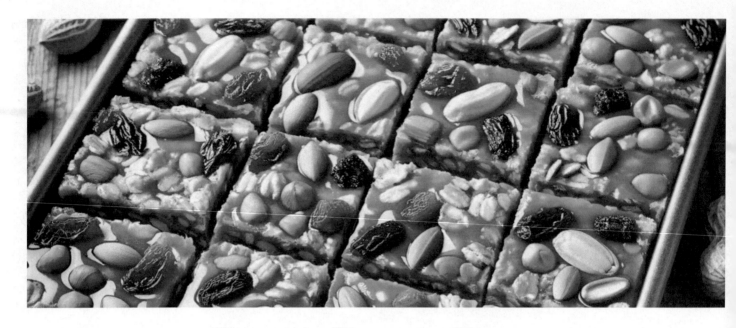

Peanut Energy Bars

Ingredients

- 1/2 cup dry roasted salted peanuts
- 1/2 cup roasted sunflower seeds
- 2 cups raisins
- 2 cups rolled oats
- 2 cups toasted rice cereal
- 1/4 cup toasted wheat germ (optional)
- 1/2 cup peanut butter
- 1/2 cup brown sugar
- 1/2 cup light corn syrup (or honey)
- 1 tsp vanilla extract

Directions

1.Prepare Pan: Coat a 9x13-inch pan with cooking spray.

2.Combine Dry Ingredients: In a large bowl, mix peanuts, seeds, raisins, oats, cereal, and wheat germ.

3.Make Syrup: In a microwaveable bowl, combine peanut butter, brown sugar, and corn syrup. Microwave on high until bubbling (1-2 minutes). Stir in vanilla.

Assemble Bars: Pour the syrup over the dry ingredients and mix well. Press into the prepared pan and let it stand for 1 hour to harden. Cut into bars.

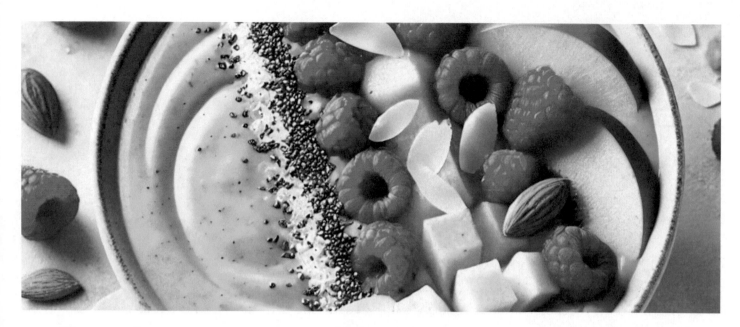

Raspberry-Peach-Mango Smoothie Bowl

Ingredients

- 1 cup frozen mango chunks
- 3/4 cup nonfat plain Greek yogurt
- 1/4 cup reduced-fat milk
- 1 tsp vanilla extract
- 1/4 ripe peach (sliced)
- 1/3 cup raspberries
- 1 tbsp sliced almonds
- 1 tbsp unsweetened coconut flakes
- 1 tsp chia seeds

Directions

1.Blend Smoothie:
In a blender, combine mango, yogurt, milk, and vanilla. Blend until smooth.

2.Assemble Bowl:
Pour the smoothie into a bowl and top with peach slices, raspberries, almonds, coconut, and chia seeds.

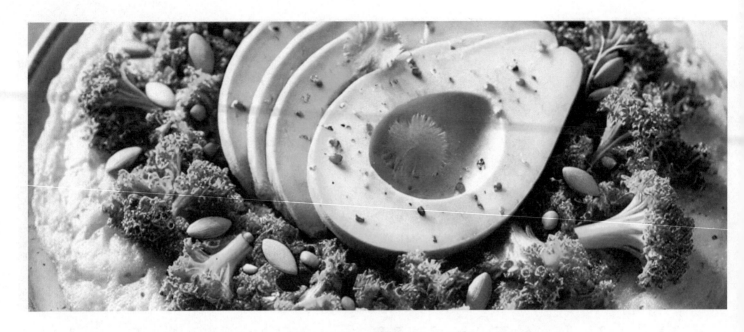

Avocado & Kale Omelet

Ingredients

- 2 large eggs
- 1 tsp low-fat milk
- Pinch of salt
- 2 tsp extra-virgin olive oil (divided)
- 1 cup chopped kale
- 1 tbsp lime juice
- 1 tbsp chopped cilantro
- 1 tsp sunflower seeds
- Pinch of crushed red pepper
- 1/4 avocado (sliced)

Directions

1.Cook Omelet:
Beat eggs with milk and salt. Heat 1 tsp oil in a skillet over medium heat. Add the eggs and cook until the bottom sets. Flip and cook for 30 seconds more. Transfer to a plate.

2.Make Salad:
Toss kale with lime juice, cilantro, sunflower seeds, red pepper, and the remaining oil. Top the omelet with kale salad and avocado.

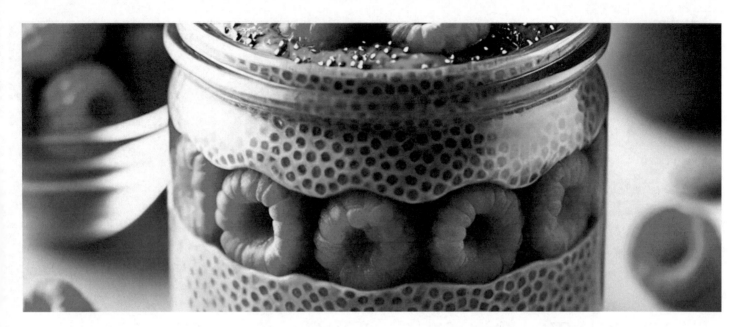

Cocoa-Chia Pudding with Raspberries

Ingredients

- 1/2 cup unsweetened almond milk
- 2 tbsp chia seeds
- 2 tsp maple syrup
- 1/2 tsp cocoa powder
- 1/4 tsp vanilla extract
- 1/2 cup fresh raspberries
- 1 tbsp toasted sliced almonds

Directions

1.Prepare Pudding:
Stir together almond milk, chia seeds, maple syrup, cocoa powder, and vanilla in a bowl. Refrigerate for at least 8 hours.
2.Assemble:
Spoon half the pudding into a bowl, top with half the raspberries and almonds, then repeat.

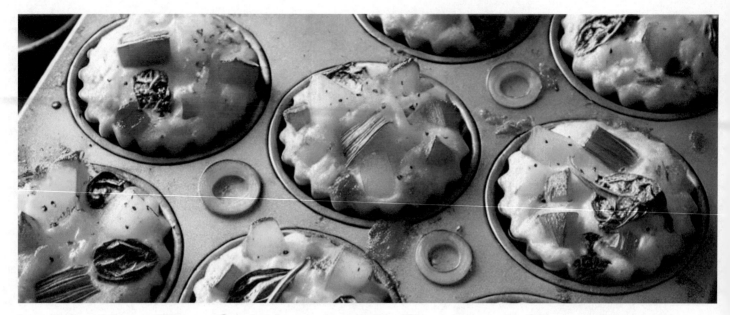

Muffin-Tin Quiches with Smoked Cheddar & Potato

Ingredients

- 2 tbsp extra-virgin olive oil
- 1 1/2 cups diced red-skinned potatoes
- 1 cup diced red onion
- 3/4 tsp salt (divided)
- 8 large eggs
- 1 cup shredded smoked cheddar cheese
- 1/2 cup low-fat milk
- 1/2 tsp ground black pepper
- 1 1/2 cups chopped fresh spinach

Directions

1.Preheat Oven: Set oven to 325°F and coat a muffin tin with cooking spray.

2.Cook Potatoes: Heat oil in a skillet over medium heat. Add potatoes, onion, and 1/4 tsp salt, cooking for 5 minutes. Let cool.

3.Mix Eggs: In a bowl, whisk together eggs, cheese, milk, pepper, and the rest of the salt. Stir in spinach and the potato mixture.

4.Bake Quiches: Divide mixture among muffin cups and bake for 25 minutes. Let cool for 5 minutes before serving.

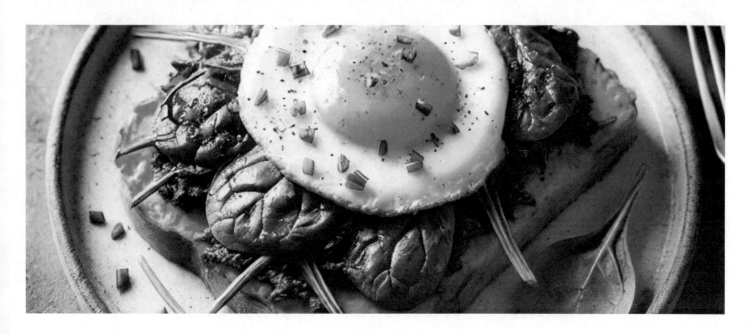

Spinach & Egg Sweet Potato Toast

Ingredients

- 1 large slice sweet potato (1/4 inch thick)
- 1/3 cup cooked spinach
- 1 large egg (fried or poached)
- 1/2 tsp fresh chives
- 1/2 tsp hot sauce

Directions

1.Toast Sweet Potato:
Toast the sweet potato in a toaster or oven until cooked through and starting to brown (12-15 minutes).
2.Assemble:
Top with spinach, egg, chives, and hot sauce.

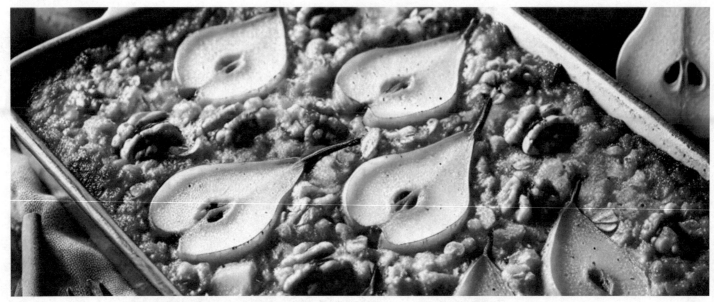

Baked Oatmeal with Pears

Ingredients

- 2 cups old-fashioned oats
- 1/2 cup walnuts (chopped)
- 2 tsp ground cinnamon
- 1 tsp baking powder
- 3/4 tsp salt
- 1/4 tsp ground nutmeg
- 1/8 tsp ground cloves
- 2 cups unsweetened almond milk (or 2% milk)
- 1 cup low-fat plain Greek yogurt (optional)
- 1/4 cup pure maple syrup
- 2 tbsp extra-virgin olive oil
- 1 tsp vanilla extract
- 2 pears (diced, about 2 cups)
- 1/3 cup low-fat plain Greek yogurt (optional for topping)

Directions

1.Preheat Oven: Preheat oven to 375°F and coat a 9-inch baking dish with cooking spray.

2.Mix Dry Ingredients: In a large bowl, mix oats, walnuts, cinnamon, baking powder, salt, nutmeg, and cloves.

3.Mix Wet Ingredients: In another bowl, whisk together the milk, 1 cup yogurt, maple syrup, olive oil, and vanilla.

4.Combine and Add Pears: Pour the wet ingredients into the dry ingredients and gently mix in the pears.

5.Bake: Transfer the mixture to the prepared dish and bake for 45-55 minutes until golden brown. Optional: Top each serving with 1 tbsp of yogurt before serving.

Tips:

- Use gluten-free oats if needed.
- Ripe pears will soften more, while unripe pears hold their shape better.
- To make ahead, store in the fridge for up to 3 days or freeze for 2 weeks.

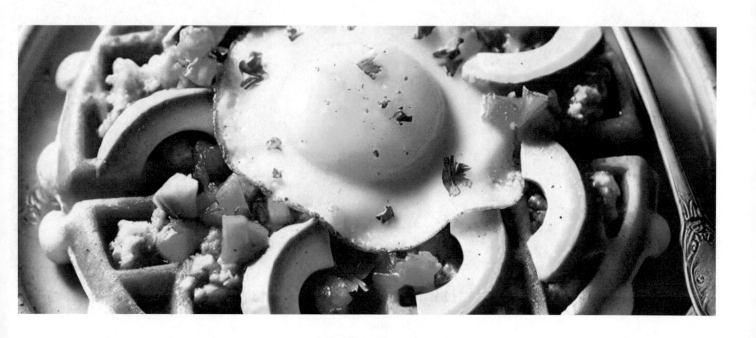

Southwestern Waffle

Ingredients

- 1 frozen whole-grain waffle
- 1 egg (cooked sunny-side up)
- 1/4 avocado (chopped)
- 1 tbsp fresh salsa

Directions

1.Toast Waffle: Toast the waffle according to the package directions.

Assemble: Top the waffle with the cooked egg, chopped avocado, and salsa.

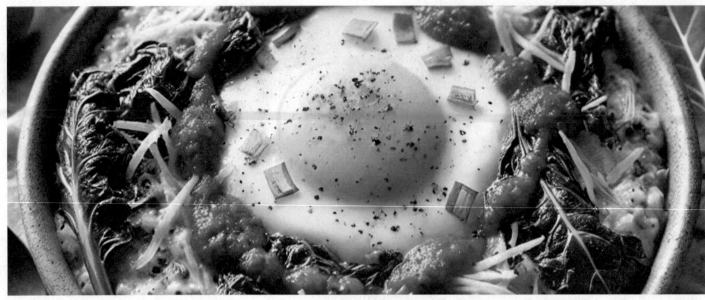

Savory Oatmeal with Cheddar, Collards & Eggs

Ingredients

- 2 tbsp extra-virgin olive oil (divided)
- 2 tbsp diced shallot
- 2 cups rolled oats
- 4 1/2 cups water (divided)
- 1/2 tsp salt (divided)
- 1/2 tsp ground pepper (divided)
- 10 cups chopped collard greens
- 2 tsp red-wine vinegar
- 1 cup shredded Cheddar cheese
- 1/4 cup chipotle salsa (plus more for serving)
- 4 large eggs (cooked as desired)

Directions

1.Cook Oats: Heat 1 tbsp oil in a saucepan over medium heat. Add shallot and cook for 1-2 minutes. Stir in oats for 1 minute. Add 4 cups water, 1/4 tsp salt, and pepper. Cook, stirring, for 10-12 minutes until creamy.

2.Cook Collards: Meanwhile, heat the remaining oil in a skillet over medium heat. Add collards, 1/2 cup water, and the remaining salt and pepper. Cook for 5-7 minutes until tender. Stir in vinegar.

3.Assemble: Stir cheese and salsa into the oatmeal. Serve with collards, eggs, and more salsa.

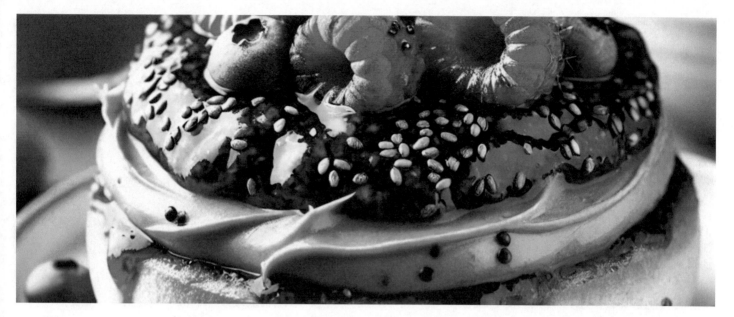

Peanut Butter & Chia Berry Jam English Muffin

Ingredients

- 1/2 cup frozen mixed berries
- 2 tsp chia seeds
- 2 tsp natural peanut butter
- 1 whole-wheat English muffin (toasted)

Directions

1.Make Jam: Microwave berries in a bowl for 30 seconds, stir, and microwave for another 30 seconds. Stir in chia seeds.

Assemble: Spread peanut butter on the toasted muffin and top with the chia berry mixture.

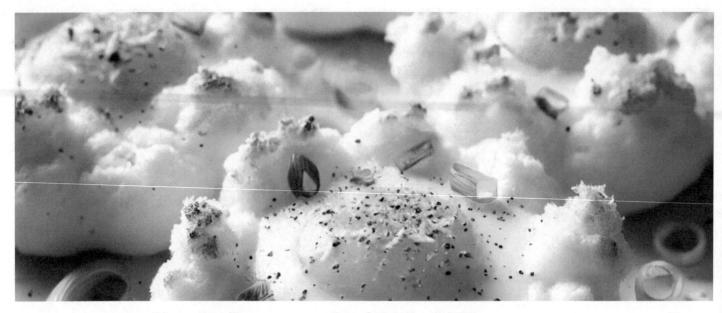

Parmesan Cloud Eggs

Ingredients

- 4 large eggs
- Pinch of salt
- 1/4 cup grated Parmesan cheese
- 1 scallion (finely chopped)
- Ground pepper (to taste)

Directions

1. Preheat Oven: Preheat oven to 450°F and line a baking sheet with parchment paper. Lightly coat with cooking spray.
2. Prepare Egg Whites: Separate the egg whites from the yolks. Beat the egg whites with salt until stiff peaks form. Fold in Parmesan and scallions.
3. Bake: Spoon the egg whites onto the baking sheet into four mounds. Make a small well in the center. Bake for 3 minutes.

Add Yolks: Gently add a yolk to each well and bake for another 3-5 minutes. Sprinkle with pepper and serve.

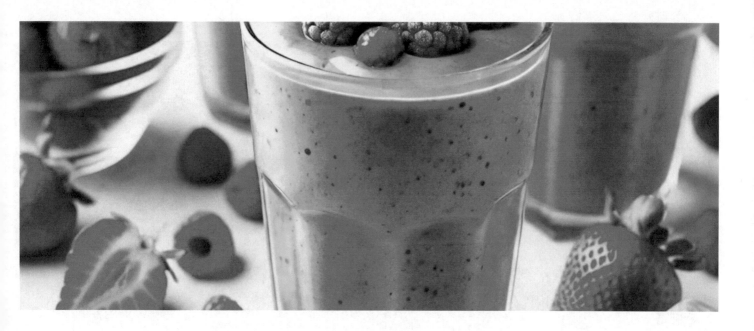

Red Berry Smoothies

Ingredients

- 1 (6 oz) container fat-free strawberry yogurt
- 1 cup fat-free milk
- 1 1/2 cups fresh strawberries (sliced)
- 1/2 cup fresh raspberries
- 1 cup ice cubes

Directions

1.Blend: In a blender, combine yogurt, milk, and fruit. Blend until smooth.
2.Add Ice: Add ice and blend again until smooth.

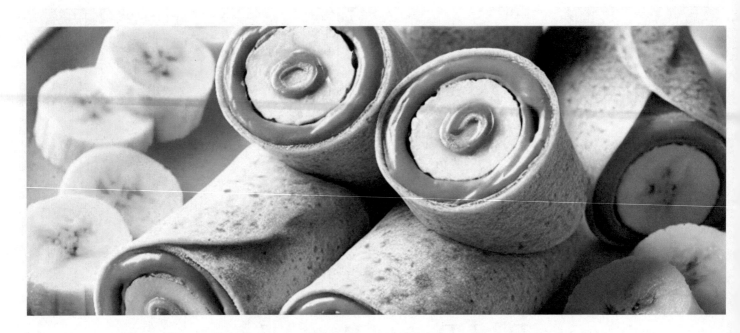

Peanut Butter-Banana Roll-Ups

Directions

Ingredients

- 2 tbsp smooth natural peanut butter (or sunflower seed butter)
- 1 tsp honey
- 1 8-inch whole-wheat tortilla
- 1 medium banana (peeled)

1.Spread: Combine peanut butter and honey, then spread evenly over the tortilla.

2.Assemble: Place the banana on the tortilla and roll tightly. Slice into 8 pieces.

Lunch Recipes

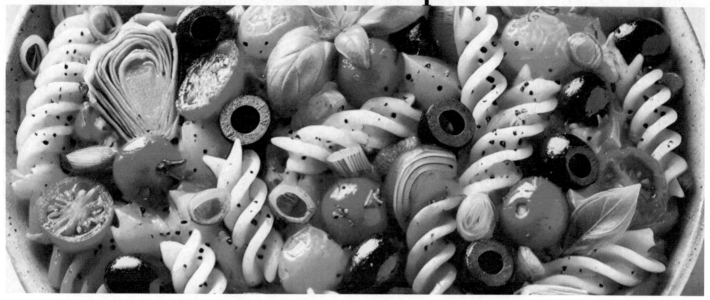

Healthy Italian Pasta Salad Recipe

Ingredients

- 1 (16 oz) box fusilli (gluten-free if desired)
- 1 clove garlic (minced)
- 1/2 cup extra-virgin olive oil
- 1/4 cup + 2 tbsp red wine vinegar
- 1 tsp Dijon mustard
- 1 tsp dried Italian seasoning
- 1 1/2 tsp salt
- 1/2 tsp pepper
- 1 (14 oz) can quartered artichoke hearts (drained)
- 1 (12 oz) jar roasted red peppers (drained and chopped)
- 1 cup chopped scallions
- 1 cup cherry tomatoes (halved)
- 1/2 cup black olives (pitted and chopped)
- 1/2 cup fresh basil (chopped)

Directions

1. Cook Pasta: Cook pasta according to package instructions until al dente (about 12 minutes). Drain.
2. Make Dressing: While pasta cooks, whisk garlic, olive oil, vinegar, mustard, Italian seasoning, salt, and pepper in a large bowl.
3. Toss Pasta: Add hot pasta to the dressing, toss to coat, and let it cool for at least 20 minutes.
4. Add Vegetables: Stir in artichokes, roasted peppers, scallions, tomatoes, olives, and basil. Serve immediately or chill.

Notes:
- The dressing can be made up to 5 days in advance.
- The recipe can be prepped up to 12 hours ahead.

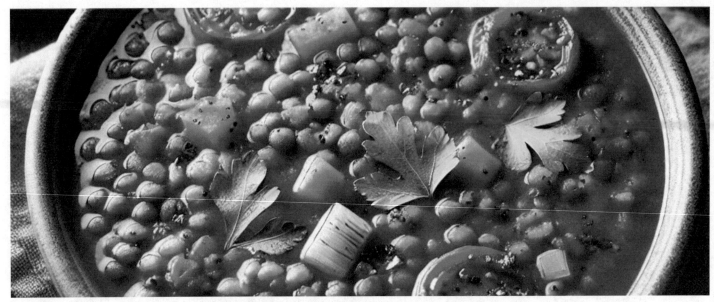

Crockpot Lentil Soup

Ingredients

- 1/2 lb dried lentils (about 1 cup + 2 tbsp)
- 1 medium yellow onion (diced)
- 2 medium carrots (diced)
- 2 celery stalks (diced)
- 2 tsp minced garlic
- 1 chipotle pepper in adobo sauce + 1 tbsp sauce (minced)
- 1 tsp ground cumin
- 1/2 tsp kosher salt (plus more to taste)
- 1/2 tsp dried oregano
- 1 (14 oz) can fire-roasted diced tomatoes
- 5 cups broth (vegetable or chicken)
- 1 bay leaf
- 2 tbsp olive oil
- 2 tsp white wine vinegar

Directions

1. Slow Cook: Add all ingredients except olive oil and vinegar to a slow cooker. Cook on low for 7-8 hours or on high for 5-6 hours.
2. Blend Soup: Remove the bay leaf. Ladle about 4 cups of the soup into a blender, add olive oil, and pulse until semi-smooth.
3. Finish Soup: Pour blended soup back into the slow cooker, stir in white wine vinegar, and season with more salt if needed.
4. Serve: Serve with toppings like cilantro, sour cream, or crusty bread.

Notes:

- If too thick, add more broth to reach the desired consistency.
- For extra spice, double the chipotle peppers.

56

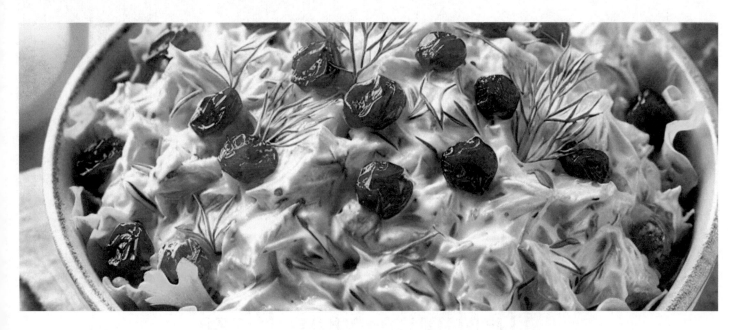

Healthy Tuna Salad with Cranberries

Ingredients

- 1 can tuna (drained)
- 2 tbsp mayonnaise
- 1 tbsp spicy brown mustard
- 1/2 tsp lemon juice
- 1/2 tsp dried oregano
- 1 tbsp chopped dill
- 2 tbsp dried cranberries

Directions

1.Flake Tuna: Flake the tuna in a medium bowl until no large chunks remain.
2.Mix: Add the remaining ingredients and mix until well combined. Serve on bread, lettuce, or eat straight from the bowl.

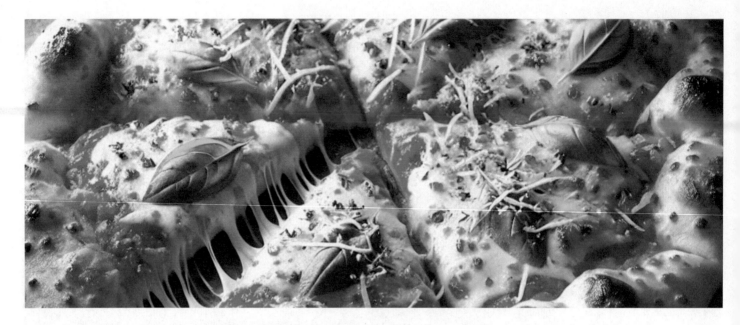

10-Minute Naan Pizza

Ingredients

- 4 naan bread pieces
- 1/2 cup pizza sauce
- 1 cup mozzarella cheese (shredded or sliced)
- 1/4 cup parmesan cheese (optional)
- 2 tbsp fresh basil (chopped)

Directions

1.Preheat Oven: Preheat oven to 425°F.

2.Assemble Pizza: Spread pizza sauce evenly over naan bread. Top with mozzarella and parmesan cheese.

3.Bake: Bake directly on the oven rack for 8-10 minutes until the crust and cheese are golden brown.

4.Serve: Slice and serve with fresh basil, parmesan, or red pepper flakes.

Notes:

- For crispier crust, pre-bake naan for 3-4 minutes before adding toppings.

For a healthier version, use whole wheat naan.

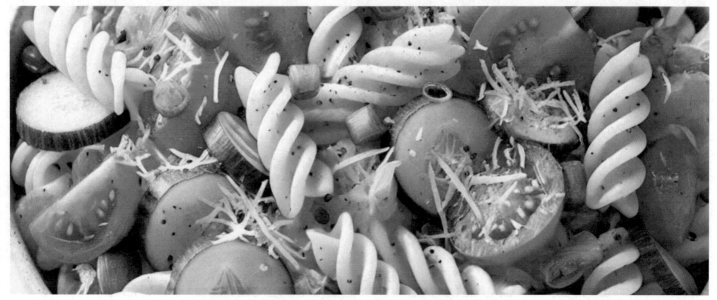

Simple Pasta Salad

Ingredients

- 1 (16 oz) package uncooked rotini pasta
- 1 (16 oz) bottle Italian salad dressing
- 2 cucumbers (chopped)
- 6 tomatoes (chopped)
- 1 bunch green onions (chopped)
- 4 oz grated Parmesan cheese
- 1 tbsp Italian seasoning

Directions

1.Cook Pasta: Cook pasta in salted water for 8-12 minutes until al dente. Drain.

2.Toss Salad: In a large bowl, toss pasta with dressing, cucumbers, tomatoes, and green onions.

3.Add Parmesan: Mix Parmesan cheese and Italian seasoning into the salad.

4.Chill: Cover and refrigerate for at least 30 minutes before serving.

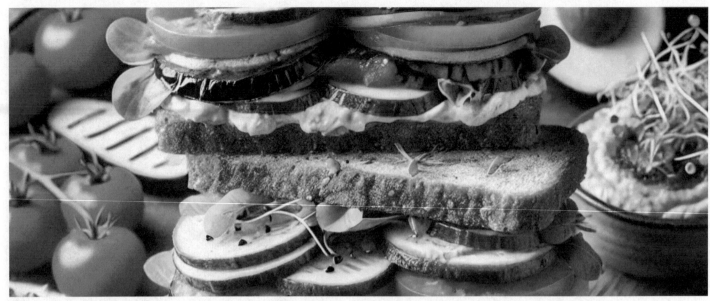

Fully-Loaded Veggie Sandwiches

Ingredients

- 1 small eggplant (or 8 portobello mushroom caps)
- 1 1/2 tbsp olive oil (or 3 tbsp for portobellos)
- Kosher salt and pepper
- 2 ripe avocados
- 2 tbsp fresh lemon juice
- 1/4 tsp red pepper flakes
- 8 slices whole-grain bread (toasted)
- 1 cup hummus (divided)
- 2 cups baby arugula (divided)
- 1 large heirloom tomato (sliced)
- 1/2 large English cucumber (sliced thin)
- 2 cups sprouts (such as broccoli or sunflower)

Directions

1.Broil Veggies: Brush eggplant or mushrooms with oil, season with salt and pepper, and broil for 4-7 minutes until tender.

2.Mash Avocado: In a bowl, mash avocado with lemon juice, red pepper flakes, and salt. Assemble Sandwiches: Spread avocado on 4 slices of toast, hummus on the remaining 4 slices then layer with arugula, tomato, cucumber, and sprouts. Assemble sandwiches.

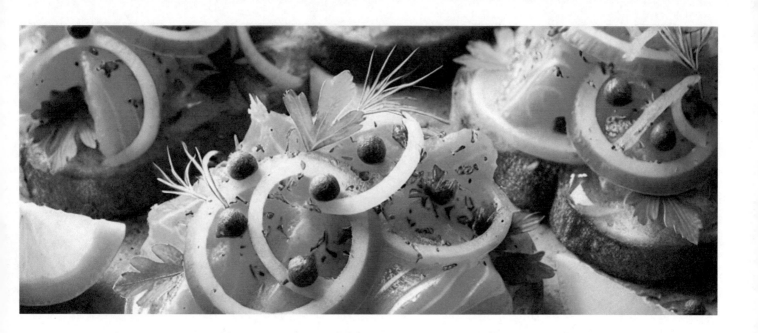

Salmon Salad Tartines

Ingredients

- 1/2 small Vidalia onion (thinly sliced)
- 1/2 bulb fennel (thinly sliced)
- 1/2 cup parsley leaves (chopped)
- 2 tbsp capers (chopped)
- 2 tbsp olive oil
- 1 tsp lemon zest + 1/2 tbsp lemon juice
- 2 (7.5 oz) cans sockeye salmon (drained)
- 4 slices sourdough bread (toasted)

Directions

1.Soak Onions: Soak sliced onion in ice water for 10 minutes, then drain and squeeze dry.

2.Mix Salad: In a bowl, combine fennel, parsley, capers, olive oil, lemon zest, and juice. Toss with onions.

3.Serve: Fold in the salmon and serve on toasted sourdough bread.

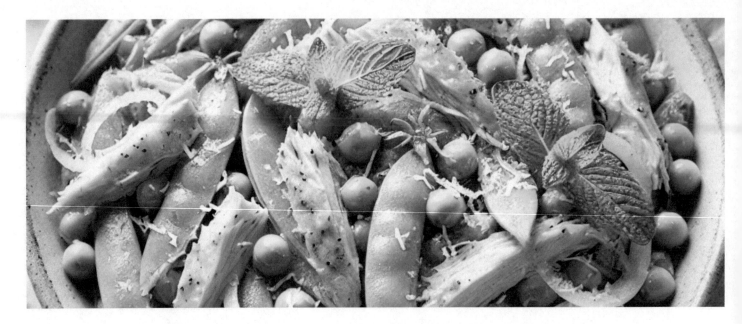

Snap Pea and Chicken Salad

Ingredients

- 1/4 cup olive oil
- 1 tsp lemon zest + 3 tbsp lemon juice
- Kosher salt and pepper
- 12 oz snap peas (thinly sliced lengthwise)
- 3 cups shredded rotisserie chicken
- 1/4 white onion (thinly sliced)
- 1/2 cup mint leaves
- 1/2 cup flat-leaf parsley leaves
- 1 oz Parmesan cheese (grated, about 1/4 cup)

Directions

1. Mix Dressing: In a large bowl, combine olive oil, lemon zest, lemon juice, 3/4 tsp salt, and 1/4 tsp pepper.
2. Toss Salad: Add snap peas, chicken, and onion to the bowl. Toss to combine.
3. Add Herbs: Fold in mint, parsley, and Parmesan. Serve immediately.

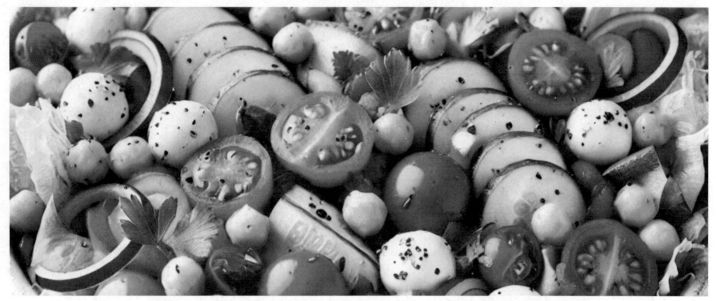

Vegetarian Antipasto Salad

Ingredients

- 2 tbsp red wine vinegar
- 2 tsp lemon zest
- 2 tbsp lemon juice
- 6 pepperoncini (chopped) + 2 tbsp pickling liquid
- 1 tbsp dried oregano
- 2 tsp Dijon mustard
- 1 small clove garlic (grated)
- Kosher salt and pepper
- 1/3 cup olive oil
- 1 small red onion (finely chopped)
- 1 (15 oz) can chickpeas (rinsed)
- 1 pint grape tomatoes (halved)
- 1/2 cup extra-small mozzarella balls (perlini)
- 2 ribs celery (thinly sliced)
- 1/2 English cucumber (cut into 1/4-inch pieces)
- 1/2 head iceberg lettuce (chopped)
- 1/2 head radicchio (chopped)
- 1/2 cup flat-leaf parsley (roughly chopped)

Directions

1. Make Dressing: In a large bowl, whisk vinegar, lemon zest, juice, pepperoncini pickling liquid, oregano, mustard, garlic, and 1/2 tsp each salt and pepper. Whisk in olive oil.
2. Toss Veggies: Stir in onion and pepperoncini and let sit for 5 minutes. Add chickpeas, tomatoes, mozzarella, celery, and cucumber. Toss to combine.
3. Assemble Salad: Toss with lettuce, radicchio, and parsley. Serve immediately or chill.

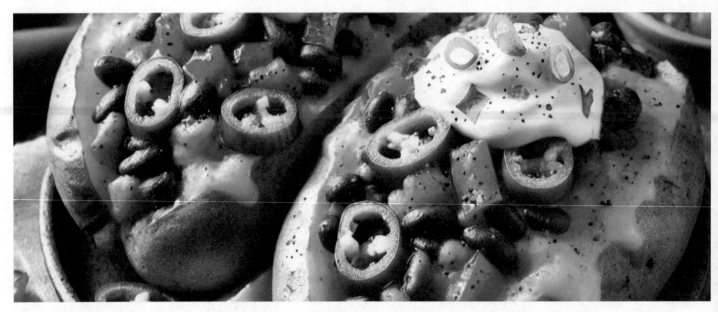

Poblano and Black Bean Loaded Baked Potato

Ingredients

- 4 medium russet potatoes (about 8 oz each)
- Olive oil
- Kosher salt
- 2 poblano peppers (cut into small pieces)
- 1 (15.5 oz) can black beans (including liquid)
- 1/2 tsp ground cumin
- 1/4 tsp smoked paprika
- 1/3 cup sour cream
- 1/2 tsp lime zest + 2 tsp lime juice
- 1 large plum tomato (seeded and chopped)
- Grated Cheddar (for serving)

Directions

1. Bake Potatoes: Preheat oven to 400°F. Prick potatoes and microwave for 10 minutes. Brush with 1 tbsp oil, sprinkle with salt, and bake for 18-20 minutes until tender.

2. Cook Peppers: Heat 1 tbsp oil in a skillet over medium heat. Add poblano peppers and cook for 5-7 minutes until tender. Transfer to a plate.

3. Prepare Beans: In the same skillet, add black beans, cumin, smoked paprika, and 1/4 tsp salt. Cook for 4-5 minutes until beans thicken. Fold in cooked poblanos.

4. Prepare Toppings: In one bowl, combine sour cream and lime zest. In another bowl, toss chopped tomato with lime juice and a pinch of salt.

5. Assemble: Split potatoes, top with cheese, beans, tomatoes, and sour cream. Sprinkle with additional lime zest if desired.

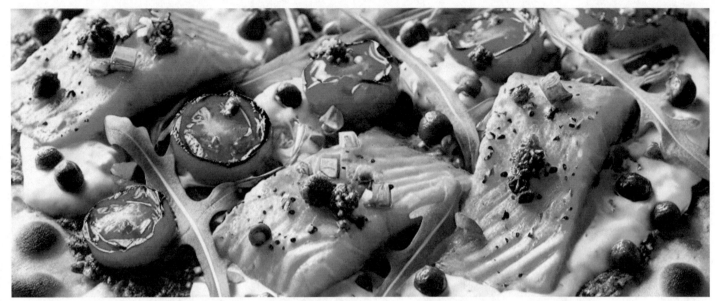

Air Fryer Salmon Flatbreads

Ingredients

- 1 tbsp red wine vinegar
- 2 tbsp olive oil (divided)
- 1 tbsp capers (chopped)
- 2 scallions (1 finely chopped, 1 thinly sliced)
- Kosher salt and pepper
- 1 pint grape tomatoes
- 1 lb skinless salmon fillet (cut into 1 1/2 inch pieces)
- 1 tbsp chopped flat-leaf parsley
- Labneh or Greek yogurt (for serving)
- 4 pieces naan or flatbread (warmed)
- 2 cups baby arugula or kale
- Crumbled feta (optional)

Directions

1.Prepare Dressing: In a small bowl, combine vinegar, 1 tbsp olive oil, capers, chopped scallion, and 1/4 tsp pepper.

2.Air-Fry Salmon and Tomatoes: Preheat air fryer to 400°F. Toss tomatoes with remaining olive oil, salt, and pepper. Season salmon with salt and pepper. Air-fry salmon and tomatoes for 6 minutes until cooked through.

3.Assemble Flatbreads: Toss tomatoes with the vinegar-scallion mixture and parsley. Spread labneh or yogurt on flatbreads, top with salmon and arugula, and spoon tomato mixture over. Garnish with sliced scallions and feta if desired.

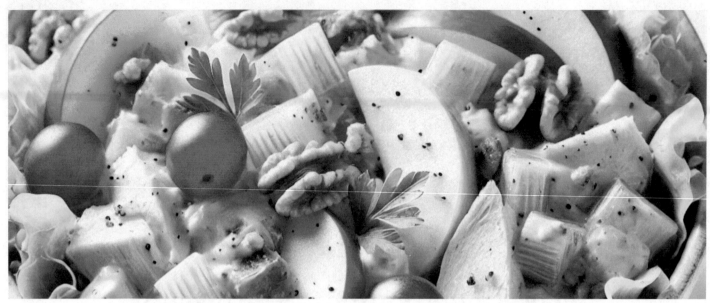

Waldorf Chicken Salad

Ingredients

- 1 tbsp white wine vinegar
- 1/2 tsp honey
- Kosher salt and pepper
- 3 tbsp sour cream
- 2 tbsp mayonnaise
- 1 tbsp whole-grain mustard
- 2 heads Boston lettuce (leaves separated)
- 3/4 cup flat-leaf parsley (roughly chopped)
- 2 rotisserie chicken breasts (sliced)
- 1 Gala apple (cored and thinly sliced)
- 2 stalks celery (thinly sliced)
- 1 cup small red grapes (halved)
- 1/2 cup walnuts (toasted and chopped)

Directions

1. Make Dressing: In a large bowl, whisk vinegar, honey, and salt. Whisk in sour cream, mayonnaise, mustard, and 1/4 tsp pepper.
2. Toss Salad: Toss lettuce with half the dressing, then add parsley. Divide among bowls, top with chicken, apple, celery, and grapes. Drizzle with remaining dressing and sprinkle with walnuts.

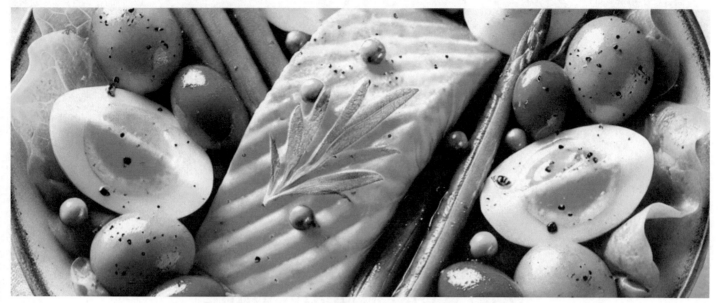

Salmon Niçoise Salad

Ingredients

- 2 tbsp olive oil
- 1 tbsp fresh lemon juice
- Kosher salt and pepper
- 1 small head green leaf lettuce (torn)
- 8 oz boiled new potatoes
- 8 oz blanched green beans
- 2 large medium-boiled eggs (halved)
- 1/4 cup kalamata olives (halved)
- 4 (5 oz) fillets cooked salmon

Directions

1.Make Dressing: In a small jar or bowl, whisk olive oil, lemon juice, and 1/4 tsp each salt and pepper.

2.Assemble Salad: Divide lettuce, potatoes, green beans, eggs, and olives among 4 bowls or food storage containers. Top with cooked salmon and drizzle with vinaigrette when ready to serve.

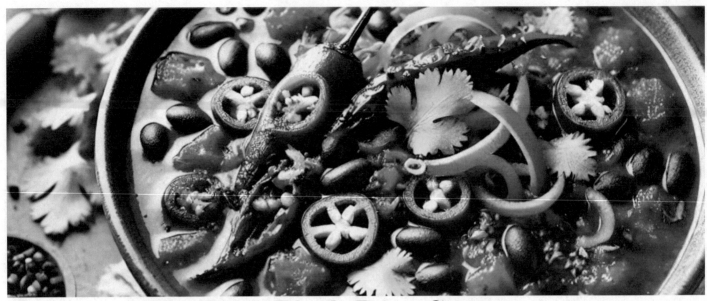

Fiery Black Bean Soup

Ingredients

Servings:

4 servings

Total Time:

45 minutes

Calories per Serving:

325

Ingredients

For the Vegetables:

- 1/2 lb. tomatillos (about 4), halved
- 2 cloves unpeeled garlic
- 1 large onion, cut into 1-inch-thick wedges
- 1 large poblano pepper, halved and seeds removed
- 1 jalapeño, halved and seeds removed
- 1 tablespoon olive oil
- Kosher salt
- Pepper

For the Soup:

- 1/2 teaspoon ground cumin
- 1/2 teaspoon ground coriander
- 4 cups low-sodium chicken broth
- 2 cans (15 oz each) low-sodium black beans, rinsed
- 1 can (14.5 oz) fire-roasted diced tomatoes, drained
- 1 small red onion, thinly sliced
- 2 tablespoons fresh lime juice
- Cilantro leaves for serving

Directions

Step 1: Prepare the Vegetables

1.Preheat the broiler.

2.On a large baking sheet, toss the tomatillos, garlic, onion, poblano pepper, and jalapeño with olive oil, 1/2 teaspoon of salt, and 1/2 teaspoon of pepper.

3.Place the peppers cut side down. Broil, turning the pan every 5 minutes, until the vegetables are soft and charred (about 15 minutes).

Step 2: Make the Soup

1.Remove the skins from the poblano peppers and garlic.

2.Finely chop all the vegetables and put them into a large pot or Dutch oven.

3.Add cumin and coriander, and cook on medium heat, stirring occasionally for about 2 minutes.

4.Pour in the chicken broth, black beans, and diced tomatoes. Bring to a simmer and let it cook for 4 minutes.

Step 3: Pickle the Red Onion

1.While the soup is cooking, mix the sliced red onion with lime juice and a pinch of salt and pepper.

2.Let the onion sit for at least 10 minutes to pickle.

Step 4: Serve

- Serve the soup in bowls and top with the pickled onion and fresh cilantro leaves.

Tip:

You can make a double batch of this soup and freeze half in small containers for up to 2 months. To reheat, thaw in the fridge overnight and then warm in a pot over medium heat. Make the pickled onions fresh just before serving.

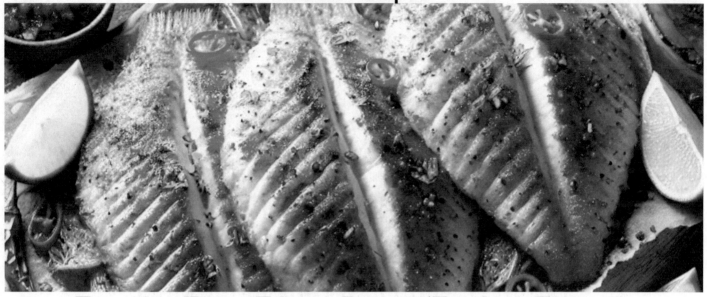

Easy Air Fryer Tilapia Recipe (Fresh or Frozen!)

Ingredients

Prep Time: 5 minutes

Cook Time: 10 minutes

Course: Main Course

Cuisine: Mexican

Servings: 2 servings

Calories: 178 kcal

Ingredients

- 12 oz tilapia fillets (6-8 oz each)
- 2 teaspoons chili powder
- 1 teaspoon cumin
- 1 teaspoon garlic powder
- 1/2 teaspoon oregano
- 1/2 teaspoon sea salt
- 1/4 teaspoon black pepper
- Zest of 1 lime
- Juice of 1/2 lime

Directions

Air Fryer Method:

1. Preheat your air fryer to 400°F if needed. Grease the air fryer basket or tray.
2. Pat the tilapia fillets dry with a paper towel.
3. Mix all the spices (except lime juice) in a small bowl.
4. Press the spice mixture into the fish on all sides.
5. Place the fillets in the air fryer, making sure they don't touch. Cook for 8-10 minutes until the fish flakes easily with a fork.
6. Drizzle with lime juice and serve right away.

Oven Method:

1. Preheat your oven to 400°F and grease a baking sheet.
2. Pat the tilapia fillets dry with a paper towel.
3. Mix all the spices (except lime juice) in a small bowl.
4. Press the spice mixture into the fish on all sides.
5. Place the fillets on the prepared baking sheet and bake for 12-14 minutes until the fish flakes easily with a fork.
6. Drizzle with lime juice and serve immediately.

Serving Tips

This air fryer tilapia has bold Mexican flavors, so it pairs well with:

- Fish tacos
- Burrito bowls
- Salads
- Rice or cauliflower rice
- Cooked plantains
- Salsa or mango salsa
- Roasted vegetables

Storage Tips

- Leftovers: Store in an airtight container for up to 4 days.
- Freezing: Store cooled, cooked tilapia in a freezer-safe container for up to 4 months. Thaw in the fridge before reheating.
- Reheating: Reheat using the same cooking method, either in the air fryer or oven, at the same temperature for up to 10 minutes.

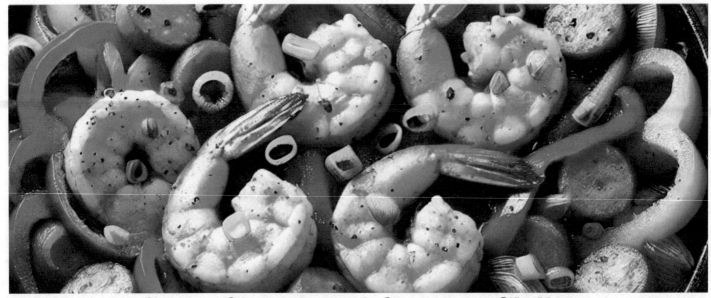

Cajun Shrimp and Sausage Skillet

Ingredients

Prep Time: 10 minutes

Cook Time: 10 minutes

Total Time: 20 minutes

Yield: 4 servings

Diet: Gluten-Free

- 2 tablespoons avocado oil or ghee
- 12 oz andouille sausage (sliced)
- 1 tablespoon minced garlic
- 1 small red bell pepper (sliced)
- 1 small green bell pepper (sliced)
- 1 small orange bell pepper (sliced)
- 1/2 yellow onion (sliced)
- 1/4 cup sliced green onion
- 1 pound shrimp (peeled and deveined)
- 1/2 tablespoon Cajun seasoning (plus more to taste)
- Juice of 1 lemon
- Salt and pepper to taste

Directions

1. Heat a large skillet over medium-high heat and add the avocado oil or ghee.
2. Add the minced garlic and cook for 1 minute until fragrant.
3. Add the andouille sausage and cook for 3-4 minutes, browning both sides. Then, add the bell peppers and onions. Season with salt, pepper, and Cajun seasoning. Cook for 3-4 minutes until the veggies soften.
4. Add the shrimp and cook for 2-3 minutes until they turn pink and are cooked through.
5. Remove from heat and stir in lemon juice, green onion, and more seasoning if desired. Serve immediately.

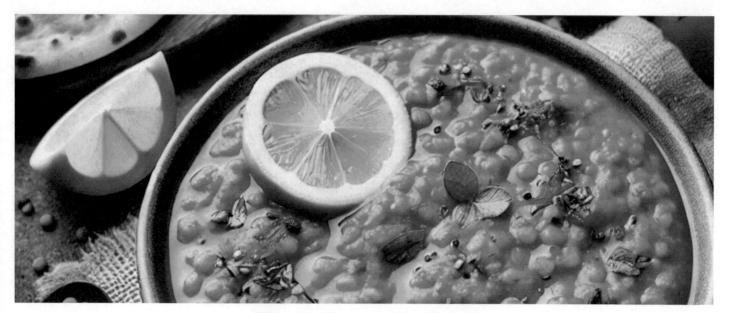

Red Lentil Dal

Ingredients

Prep Time: 10 minutes

Cook Time: 26 minutes

Total Time: 36 minutes

- 1 tbsp extra-virgin olive oil
- 1 large yellow onion, diced
- 4 cloves garlic, minced
- 1 tbsp grated fresh ginger (or ¼ tsp ground ginger)
- 1 tbsp garam masala or curry powder
- 1½ cups dried red lentils
- 3 cups low-sodium vegetable broth
- 1 (13.5-oz) can light coconut milk
- 1 (14-oz) can diced tomatoes
- ½ tsp kosher salt
- 1 lemon, cut into 8 wedges
- 4 pieces naan (preferably whole-grain), sliced in half

Directions

1.Heat a large skillet over medium heat. Add the oil and onion, cooking for about 5 minutes until soft. Stir in garlic, ginger, and garam masala, and cook for 1 more minute until fragrant.

2.Add lentils, broth, coconut milk, and tomatoes (with their juices). Turn the heat to high and bring to a boil, then lower to a simmer. Cook for about 15 minutes, stirring often, until the lentils are soft but not mushy.

3.Season with salt, and serve with a lemon wedge and naan.

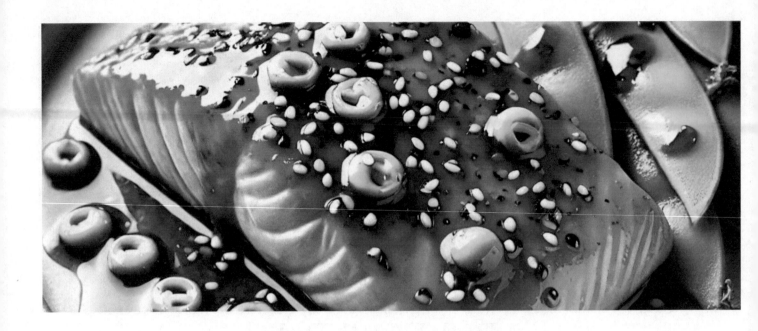

Miso Glazed Salmon with Snap Peas

Ingredients

Serves: 4

Prep Time: 3 minutes

Cook Time: 8 minutes

- 4 (6-ounce) skinless salmon fillets
- 1/4 cup white miso
- 1/4 cup maple syrup
- 1/4 cup mirin
- 1 tbsp ginger
- 1 tbsp sesame oil
- 1 cup sugar snap peas

Directions

1.In a bowl, whisk together miso, maple syrup, mirin, ginger, and sesame oil. Add the salmon and coat well.

2.Preheat the broiler and adjust the oven rack to about 6 inches from the heat. Line a baking sheet with parchment paper and place the salmon on it. Broil for 5-8 minutes until the glaze is browned and the salmon is cooked through.

3.While the salmon cooks, steam the snap peas for about 5 minutes until crisp-tender.

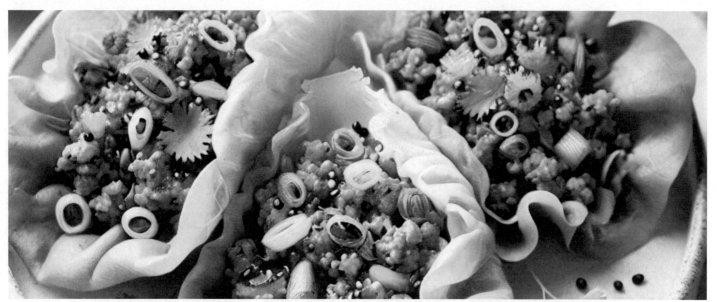

Healthy Pork Lettuce Wraps

Ingredients

Serves: 4

Prep Time: 5 minutes

Cook Time: 10 minutes

- 2 tsp vegetable oil
- 1 lb lean ground pork
- 4 green onions, thinly sliced
- 1 tsp ground allspice
- 1/2 tsp ground ginger
- 2 cloves garlic, chopped
- 2 tbsp low-sodium soy sauce (gluten-free if needed)
- 16 butter lettuce or romaine leaves
- 8 tsp plum sauce (gluten-free if needed)
- 2 tbsp chopped cilantro
- 1 lime, cut into 4 wedges

Directions

1.Heat oil in a large frying pan over high heat and cook the pork until browned. Drain excess fat.

2.Add green onions, allspice, ginger, garlic, and soy sauce. Cook for about 2 minutes until the onions are tender.

3.Place 4 lettuce leaves on each plate and fill with the pork mixture. Top with plum sauce and cilantro, and serve with a lime wedge.

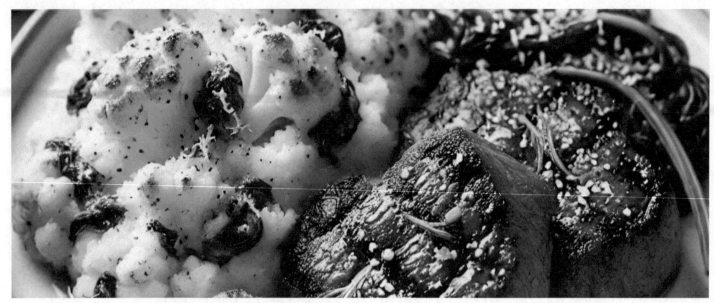

Steak and Cauliflower Potatoes with Sautéed Spinach

Ingredients

Serves: 2

Prep Time: 2 minutes

Cook Time: 20 minutes

- Cooking spray
- 2 (3.5-ounce) top sirloin steaks
- 3/4 tsp kosher salt
- 1/2 tsp black pepper
- 4 cups cauliflower florets
- 2 tbsp nonfat milk
- 2 tbsp Parmesan cheese
- 1 small garlic clove
- 6 cups spinach

Directions

1.Heat a cast iron skillet over high heat and coat with cooking spray. Pat steaks dry and season with salt and pepper. Cook for 3-6 minutes per side, depending on your desired doneness.

2.Boil cauliflower in water until tender, about 6 minutes. Drain and blend with milk, cheese, and garlic until smooth.

3.In the same skillet, sauté spinach for about 1 minute until wilted. Serve the steaks with cauliflower mash and spinach.

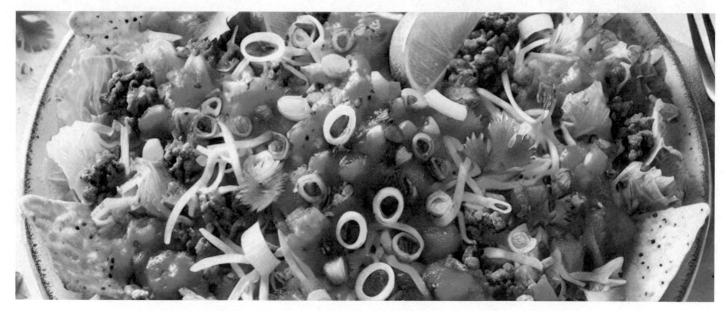

Quick and Easy Taco Salad

Ingredients

Serves: 4

Total Time: 10 minutes

- 1 lb ground beef (or turkey, 85% lean)
- 2 tsp taco seasoning
- 1/4 cup chopped cilantro
- 2 romaine lettuce hearts, chopped
- 1 cup shredded Mexican blend cheese (reduced-fat)
- 1 cup salsa
- 4 scallions, minced
- 1 cup crumbled baked corn tortilla chips (about 12 chips)
- 1 lime, cut into 4 wedges

Directions

1.Cook ground beef or turkey in a skillet over medium-high heat for about 6 minutes until browned. Stir in taco seasoning.

2.Remove from heat and sprinkle cilantro on top.

3.Divide lettuce, salsa, cheese, scallions, chips, and meat evenly among 4 plates. Serve with lime wedges.

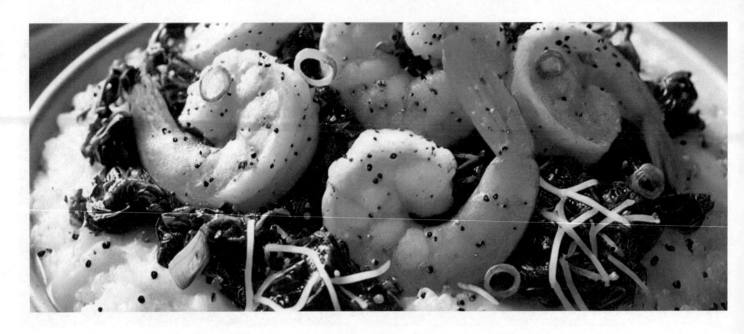

Quinoa and Shrimp Grits

Ingredients

Serves: 4

Prep Time: 5 minutes

Cook Time: 20 minutes

- 3/4 cup quinoa
- 5 oz shredded cheddar cheese
- 1 tsp vegetable oil
- 1 lb medium shrimp, peeled and deveined
- 2 tsp Cajun seasoning
- 4 cups chopped Swiss chard
- 2 tbsp water
- 1 cup nonfat plain Greek yogurt
- 4 scallions (green parts only), minced

Directions

1. Cook quinoa in 2 cups of water over low heat for 12-15 minutes until tender. Stir in cheese and set aside.

2. Heat oil in a skillet and cook shrimp with Cajun seasoning for 2-3 minutes. Set aside.

3. Add Swiss chard and water to the skillet, cooking until wilted. Stir in yogurt.

Serve quinoa topped with chard and shrimp, garnished with scallions.

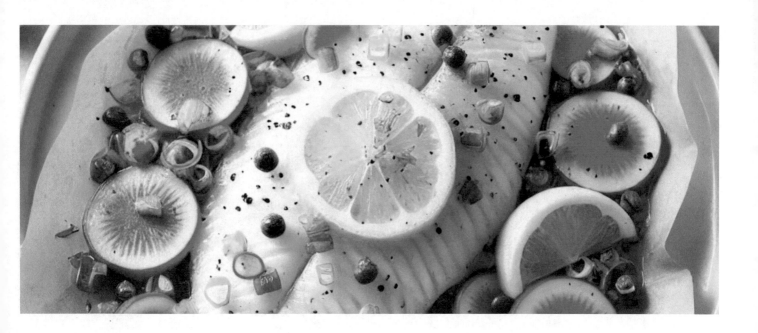

Baked Tilapia with Radish Relish

Ingredients

Serves: 4

Prep Time: 5 minutes

Cook Time: 10 minutes

- 4 (8-ounce) tilapia fillets (skinless, boneless)
- 1/8 tsp fine sea salt
- 1/8 tsp black pepper
- 1/2 lemon, thinly sliced
- 1 bunch radishes, chopped
- 1 green onion, thinly sliced
- 2 tbsp capers, chopped
- 1 tbsp lemon juice

Directions

1.Preheat the oven to 400°F. Cut parchment paper into 4 squares and fold each in half. Place a tilapia fillet on each piece of paper, season with salt, pepper, and lemon slices.

2.Fold the parchment to seal the fish, then bake for about 10 minutes until cooked through.

3.For the relish, combine radishes, green onion, capers, and lemon juice. Serve with the fish.

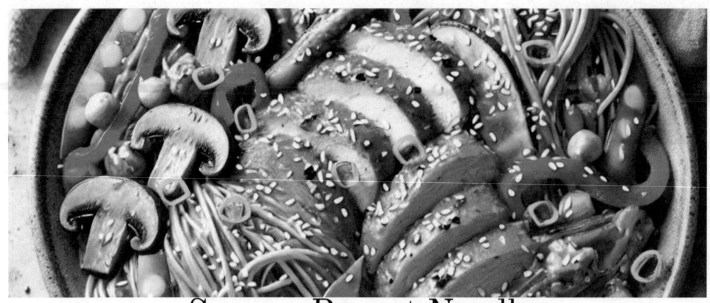

Sesame Peanut Noodles

Ingredients

Serves: 4

Prep Time: 10 minutes

Cook Time: 15 minutes

- 1/2 lb whole-wheat spaghetti
- 1 tbsp dark sesame oil
- 3/4 lb chicken breasts (cut into strips or cubes)
- 1 1/2 tbsp grated fresh ginger
- 3 cloves garlic, minced
- 3 tbsp peanut butter
- 1 tbsp sesame tahini
- 2 tbsp honey
- 2 tbsp soy sauce (reduced-sodium)
- 1 tbsp rice vinegar
- 3/4 tsp red pepper flakes
- 1 cup sliced shiitake mushrooms
- 1 red bell pepper, sliced
- 1 cup snow peas
- 1 large zucchini, sliced
- 3 scallions, sliced
- 2 tbsp toasted sesame seeds

Directions

1. Cook pasta according to package directions. Drain and rinse under cold water.

2. Heat sesame oil in a skillet, cook chicken until browned. Remove chicken and set aside.

3. Cook ginger and garlic for 1 minute, then add peanut butter, tahini, honey, soy sauce, vinegar, red pepper flakes, and pasta water. Stir until creamy.

4. Add mushrooms, bell pepper, snow peas, and zucchini, cooking for 2-3 minutes. Stir in chicken and noodles, then top with scallions and sesame seeds.

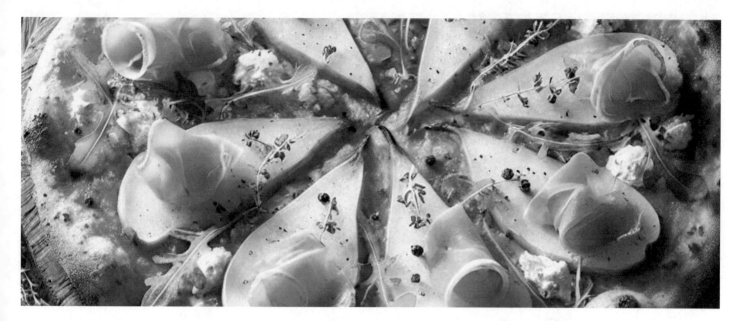

Pear and Prosciutto Pizza

Ingredients

Serves: 8

Prep Time: 8 minutes

Cook Time: 12 minutes

- 1 lb whole-wheat pizza dough
- 1 tbsp olive oil
- 4 oz low-fat goat cheese (crumbled)
- 3 cups fresh arugula
- 2 tsp chopped thyme
- 1 tsp lemon juice
- 1/2 tsp black pepper
- 3 oz thinly sliced prosciutto
- 1 ripe Bartlett pear, thinly sliced

Directions

1.Preheat the oven to 450°F. Roll out pizza dough into a 14-inch circle and transfer to a baking sheet. Brush with olive oil and sprinkle with goat cheese. Bake for 12 minutes.

2.Toss arugula with thyme, lemon juice, and black pepper.

3.Arrange prosciutto, pear, and arugula salad on the pizza. Cut into 8 slices and serve.

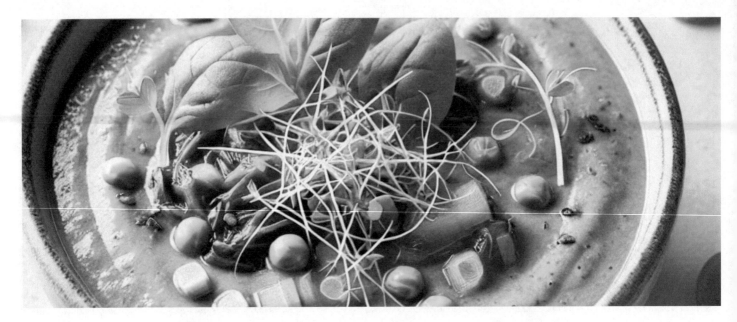

Spring Green Detox Soup

Ingredients

Serves: 4

Prep Time: 15 minutes

Cook Time: 15 minutes

- 1 tablespoon olive oil
- 2 large leeks, thinly sliced (white and green parts)
- 1 large sweet potato, peeled and cubed
- 5 cloves garlic, chopped
- 5 cups water
- 2 cups shelled fresh or frozen peas
- 4 cups baby spinach, packed
- Sea salt and pepper, to taste
- Sprouts or fresh herbs for garnish

Directions

1.Heat olive oil in a large pot over medium heat. Add leeks and a pinch of salt, sauté for 3 minutes until soft. Add sweet potato, garlic, and 4 cups of water. Bring to a boil, reduce heat, and simmer covered for 15 minutes until sweet potato is tender.

2.Remove from heat, then add peas, spinach, and 1 cup of cold water. Stir until spinach wilts and peas are vibrant.

Use an immersion blender to puree until smooth Season with salt and pepper. Serve with sprouts or fresh herbs.

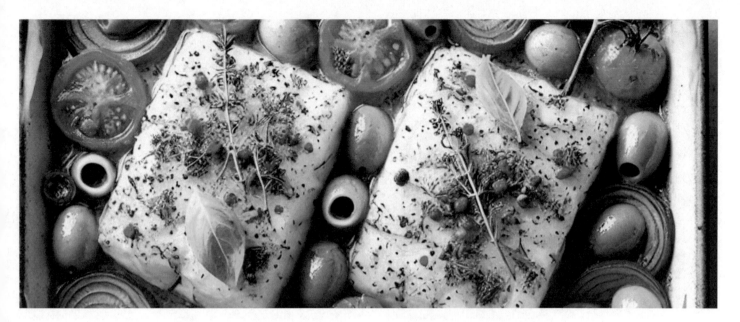

Mediterranean Baked Cod

Ingredients

Serves: 4

Prep Time: 10 minutes

Cook Time: 10 minutes

- 4 cod fillets
- 1 tablespoon olive oil
- 1 tablespoon lemon juice
- ¼ cup green olives, pitted
- ½ red onion, sliced
- 1 package cherry tomatoes, halved
- 1 teaspoon dried basil
- 1 teaspoon dried dill
- 1 teaspoon dried thyme
- ½ teaspoon salt
- ½ teaspoon black pepper
- Lemon wedges for serving (optional)

Directions

1.Preheat the oven to 400°F. Coat a baking dish with olive oil and place cod fillets in it. Drizzle with lemon juice.

2.Add olives, sliced onion, and halved cherry tomatoes around the cod.

3.Sprinkle with basil, dill, thyme, salt, and pepper.

4.Bake for 10 minutes, until cod is cooked through (internal temp 145°F). Serve with lemon wedges.

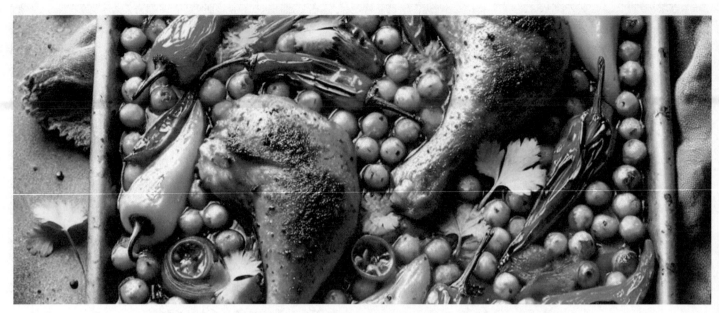

Sheet Pan Chickpea Chicken

Ingredients

Serves: 4

Total Time: 25 minutes

- 1 (15.5-oz) can chickpeas, rinsed
- 1 (16-oz) bag mini sweet peppers
- 2 tablespoons olive oil, divided
- Kosher salt and pepper
- 2 tablespoons harissa sauce
- 4 small skin-on chicken legs (about 2 1/2 pounds)
- Chopped cilantro for serving

Directions

1. Preheat oven to 425°F. Toss chickpeas and peppers with 1 tablespoon oil, salt, and pepper on a large rimmed baking sheet.
2. In a small bowl, mix harissa and 1 tablespoon oil. Rub this mixture on the chicken legs and place them among the chickpeas and peppers.
3. Roast for 20-25 minutes, until chicken is golden and cooked through. Serve with cilantro.

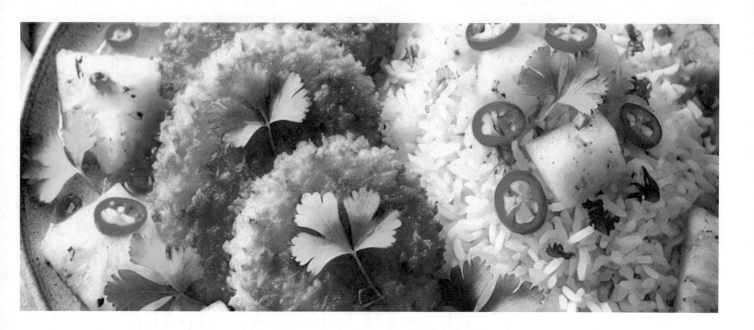

Baked Chicken Cutlets with Pineapple Rice

Ingredients

Serves: 4

Total Time: 25 minutes

- 1 cup long-grain white rice
- 1/4 cup reduced-sodium soy sauce
- 1 tablespoon rice vinegar
- 1 1/2 tablespoons grated fresh ginger
- 8 small chicken cutlets (about 1 1/4 lbs)
- 1 1/4 cups panko breadcrumbs
- 1 1/2 tablespoons canola oil
- 1 small red chili, thinly sliced
- 1/2 small pineapple, thinly sliced
- 1 cup fresh cilantro leaves

Directions

1.Preheat the oven to 450°F and line a baking sheet with nonstick foil. Cook rice according to package instructions.

2.In a bowl, mix soy sauce, vinegar, and ginger. Toss half of this mixture with the chicken.

3.Coat chicken in panko mixed with oil. Place on baking sheet and bake for 10-12 minutes until golden brown.

4.Fluff rice and toss with chili, pineapple, and cilantro. Serve chicken with rice and remaining sauce.

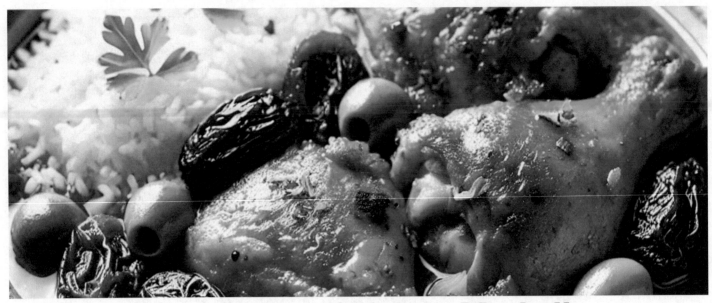

Slow Cooker Chicken Marbella

Ingredients

Serves: 4

Prep Time: 15 minutes

Total Time: 6 hours

- 1/2 cup dry white wine
- 2 tablespoons brown sugar
- 1 1/2 teaspoons dried oregano
- 3 tablespoons red wine vinegar
- Kosher salt and pepper
- 6 cloves garlic
- 1 tablespoon capers
- 1/2 cup prunes
- 1/4 cup pitted green olives
- 4 small chicken legs (split into drumsticks and thighs, about 2 1/2 lbs)
- 1/4 cup chopped parsley
- 1 cup long-grain white rice

Directions

1.In a slow cooker, whisk wine, brown sugar, oregano, 2 tablespoons vinegar, salt, and pepper. Add garlic, capers, prunes, and olives. Stir to combine.

2.Nestle chicken among olives and prunes. Cook on low for 5-6 hours (or on high for 3-4 hours).

3.Stir in remaining vinegar and parsley. Serve chicken with rice and cooking liquid.

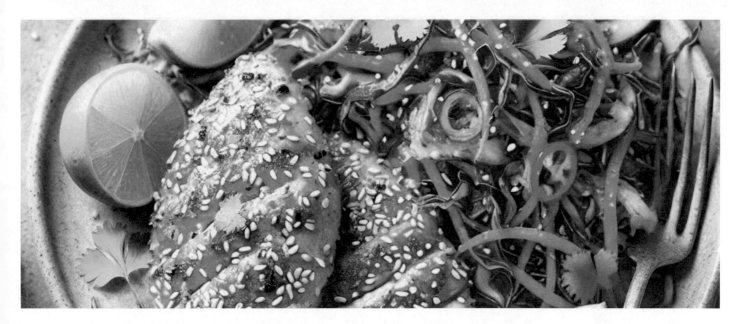

Sesame Chicken with Chili Lime Slaw

Ingredients

Serves: 4

Total Time: 20 minutes

- 2 large egg whites
- Kosher salt and pepper
- 4 boneless, skinless chicken breasts (5 oz each)
- 1/2 cup sesame seeds
- 1 tablespoon olive oil
- 1/4 cup lime juice
- 1 tablespoon grated fresh ginger
- 1 teaspoon honey
- 1 small red chili, thinly sliced
- 1/2 small head red cabbage, finely shredded
- 2 large carrots, coarsely grated
- 1/2 cup fresh cilantro leaves

Directions

1.Preheat oven to 425°F. Beat egg whites with 1/2 teaspoon salt. Dip chicken in egg whites, then coat with sesame seeds.

2.Heat oil in a skillet over medium heat. Brown chicken for 5 minutes on one side, then transfer skillet to the oven. Roast for 8-10 minutes until cooked through.

In a large bowl, mix lime juice, ginger, honey, and salt. Toss cabbage and carrots in the dressing, then fold in cilantro. Serve with chicken.

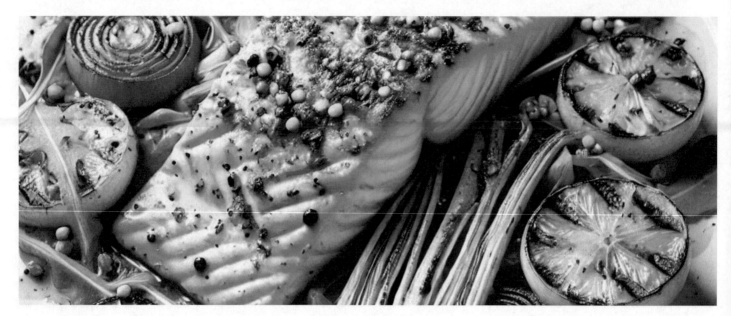

Oven-Roasted Salmon with Charred Lemon Vinaigrette

Ingredients

Serves: 4

Total Time: 35 minutes

- 1 lemon
- 2 bulbs fennel, thinly sliced
- 2 small red onions, thinly sliced
- 2 1/2 tablespoons olive oil, divided
- Kosher salt and pepper
- 1 1/4 lbs skin-on salmon fillet
- 1 teaspoon stone-ground mustard
- 3 cups baby arugula

Directions

1.Preheat broiler. Cut lemon in half and broil for 5 minutes until charred. Set aside.

2.Lower oven temperature to 400°F. Toss fennel and onions with 1 1/2 tablespoons oil, salt, and pepper. Arrange around the edges of a baking sheet and place salmon in the center. Season with salt and pepper. Roast for 17-20 minutes.

3.Juice charred lemon into a bowl, whisk in mustard and remaining oil. Remove salmon and fold arugula into roasted vegetables. Drizzle with lemon vinaigrette.

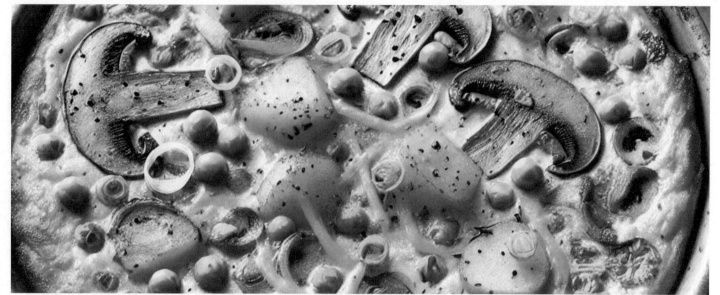

Wild Mushroom Frittata with Cheddar, Green Onions, and Peas

Ingredients

Total Time: 30 minutes

Serves: 2

- 6 large eggs
- 2 tbsp milk or water
- Salt and freshly ground black pepper
- Pinch of grated nutmeg
- Pinch of cayenne pepper
- 2 tbsp unsalted butter
- 3 new potatoes, diced
- 4 green onions, sliced
- 10 oz wild mushrooms (cremini, shiitake, oyster), cleaned and sliced
- 1 garlic clove, minced
- 1 tsp fresh thyme, minced
- 1/2 cup frozen peas, thawed
- 1/2 cup shredded Cheddar cheese

Directions

1.Preheat the broiler with the rack in the second-highest position.

2.In a bowl, whisk eggs, milk, salt, pepper, nutmeg, and cayenne.

3.In an ovenproof skillet, melt butter over medium-high heat. Add potatoes, season with salt and pepper, and cook for 3 minutes. Add green onions, mushrooms, garlic, thyme, and cook for another 4 minutes until mushrooms are dry. Add peas and cook for another 2 minutes.

4.Spread veggies evenly in the pan and sprinkle cheese on top. Pour the egg mixture over the vegetables.

Cook on low heat for 2 minutes, then broil for about 4 minutes until the top is lightly browned and eggs are set. Let the frittata rest for 3 minutes before cutting and serving.

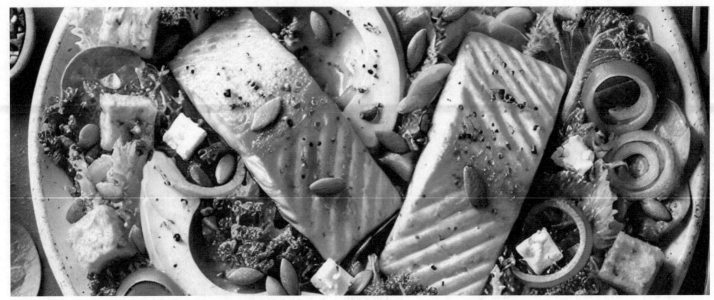

Superfood Salmon Salad

Ingredients

Total Time: 55 minutes

Servings: 2

- 2 (4 oz) salmon fillets
- 1 tbsp avocado oil
- Salt and pepper, to taste
- 4 cups baby kale and romaine or spring mix
- 2 cups sweet potato croutons
- 1/2 avocado, sliced
- 1/4 cup pickled red onions
- 1/4 cup crumbled feta
- 2 tbsp pepitas
- Lemon vinaigrette

Directions

1. Prepare pickled red onions, lemon vinaigrette, and sweet potato croutons.
2. Season salmon with salt and pepper. Heat oil in a skillet over medium-high heat. Cook salmon skin-side up for 4 minutes, then flip and cook for another 4 minutes until medium-rare.
3. Toss greens with sweet potato croutons, onions, feta, and pepitas. Divide onto two plates.
4. Top with salmon, avocado, and drizzle with vinaigrette. Season with extra salt and pepper if needed.

Notes:

- Dairy-free: Leave out the feta for a dairy-free version.
- Mix-ins: Switch up veggies based on what you have available.
- Dressing alternatives: You can use balsamic vinaigrette or another dressing in a pinch.

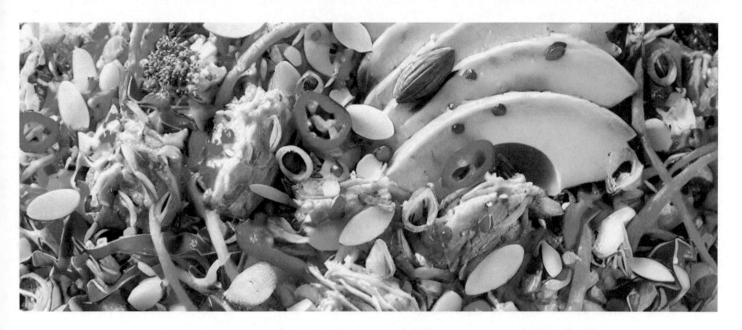

Crunchy Asian Chopped Salad

Ingredients

Total Time: 10 minutes

Servings: 2

- 3 cups napa cabbage or romaine, chopped
- 5 cups purple cabbage, chopped
- 1/2 cup shredded carrots
- 1 cup red bell pepper, chopped
- 1 avocado, sliced
- 2-3 green onions, sliced
- 1/4 cup cilantro, chopped
- 1/4 cup chopped almonds
- 2 cups shredded chicken
- Chili almond dressing

Directions

1.Toss the cabbage, carrots, bell pepper, green onions, cilantro, and chicken in a large bowl.

2.Add the dressing and toss again.

3.Portion the salad and top with avocado slices and almonds.

Notes:

- Make it vegetarian: Omit chicken and add chickpeas, tempeh, or tofu for protein.

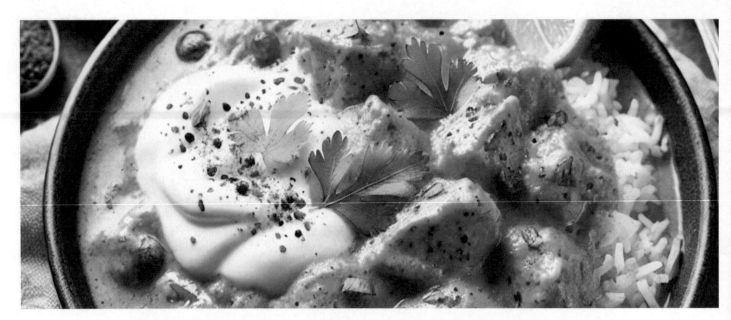

30-Minute Thai Chicken Curry

Ingredients

Total Time: 30 minutes

- 1 (14 oz) can full-fat coconut milk
- 1/2 yellow onion, finely chopped
- 1 tbsp fresh ginger, grated
- 2 tsp ground cumin
- 1 1/2 tsp ground coriander
- 1 tsp ground turmeric
- 1 tsp paprika
- 2 tsp garlic powder
- 1 tsp sea salt
- 1 lb boneless, skinless chicken breasts, chopped

For serving:

- Cooked rice
- Fresh cilantro, chopped
- Plain or Greek yogurt
- Lime wedges

Directions

1. Cook rice according to package instructions.
2. In a skillet, sauté onion and ginger with 1/3 cup coconut milk over medium-high heat for 6-8 minutes.
3. Lower the heat, add the spices, and cook for 3 more minutes. If it gets too dry, add more coconut milk.
4. Add the rest of the coconut milk and bring to a boil. Add chicken and cook for 5-6 minutes until done.

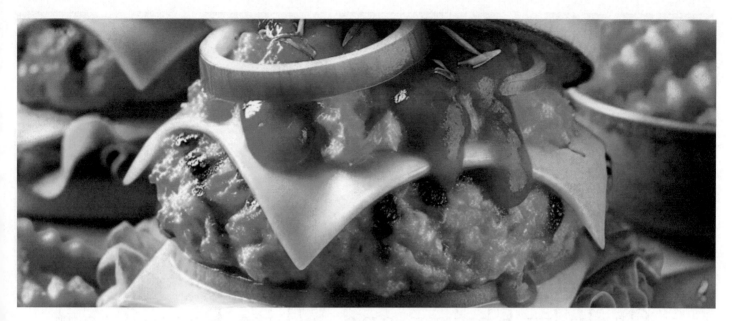

Sweet Potato Cheddar BBQ Chicken Burgers

Ingredients

Total Time: 30 minutes

Servings: 4

- 1 lb ground chicken (or turkey, 93% lean)
- 1 cup shredded sweet potato
- 2 tbsp low-sugar BBQ sauce
- 1/4 cup yellow onion, finely diced
- 2 cloves garlic, minced
- 1/2 tsp cumin
- 1/2 tsp salt
- Ground black pepper
- 4 slices sharp cheddar cheese
- 4 hamburger buns
- Lettuce and sliced red onion for serving
- Extra BBQ sauce for topping

Directions

1. In a bowl, mix chicken, sweet potato, BBQ sauce, onion, garlic, cumin, salt, and pepper. Shape into 4 patties.
2. Grill over medium-high heat for 5-8 minutes per side until fully cooked (internal temp 165°F). Add cheddar slices during the last minute to melt.
3. Serve on buns with lettuce, red onion, and extra BBQ sauce.

Notes:

- Serve with sweet potato fries or fresh fruit.

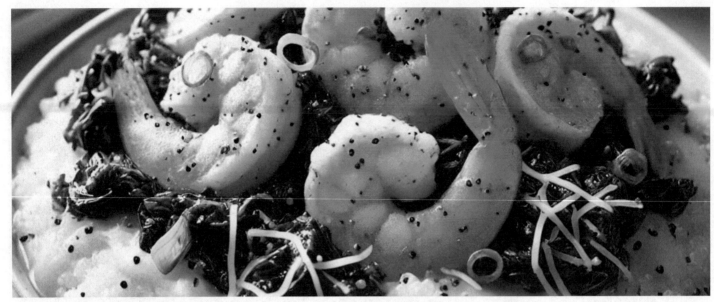

Garlicky Shrimp and White Bean Toast

Ingredients

Servings: 4

Total Time: 20 minutes

Calories per Serving: 380

- 5 tbsp olive oil, divided
- 6 cloves garlic, thinly sliced, divided
- 3 sprigs fresh thyme
- 1 lemon
- 1 cup canned white beans, rinsed
- Kosher salt and pepper
- 1 lb large shrimp, deveined, tails removed, butterflied
- 1/2 tsp red pepper flakes
- 1 bay leaf
- 1/4 cup dry sherry
- 2 cups baby spinach, roughly chopped
- 2 tbsp chopped parsley
- 4 slices of toasted bread

Directions

1.In a small skillet, heat 2 tbsp oil, half of the garlic, and thyme sprigs over medium heat for 1-2 minutes until garlic sizzles. Remove thyme, add 1 tsp lemon zest, and 1 tbsp lemon juice. Blend beans, 1/4 tsp salt and pepper in a food processor until smooth.

2.Heat remaining 3 tbsp oil in a large skillet on medium-low. Add remaining garlic, cooking for 4 minutes until golden. Add shrimp, red pepper flakes, bay leaf, and thyme. Season with salt, increase heat to medium-high, and cook for 1 minute.

3.Add sherry, reduce heat to medium-low, and cook until shrimp is opaque (1-2 minutes). Remove bay leaf, toss with spinach and parsley.

4.Spread the bean mixture on toast and top with shrimp, spinach, and pan juices.

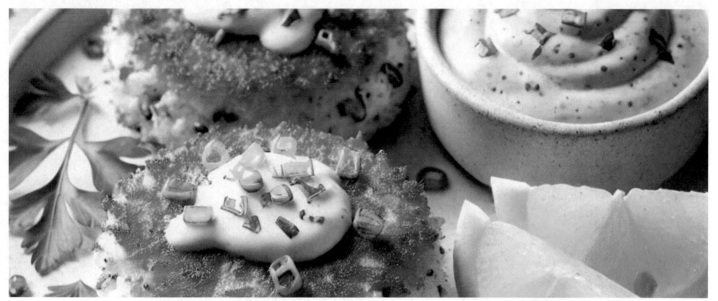

Crab Cakes and Creamy Sauce

Ingredients

Servings: 8

Total Time: 25 minutes

For the Creamy Sauce:

- 1/4 cup mayonnaise
- 1 tbsp Dijon mustard
- 1/2 tbsp whole-grain mustard
- 2 tsp lemon juice
- 1/4 tsp hot sauce (like Tabasco)
- 1 scallion, finely chopped
- 1 tbsp chopped capers or pickles (optional)

For the Crab Cakes:

- 1/3 cup mayonnaise
- 1 large egg
- 2 tbsp Dijon mustard
- 1 tsp Worcestershire sauce
- 1/4 to 1/2 tsp hot sauce
- 2 scallions, finely chopped
- 2 tbsp parsley, finely chopped
- 2 tsp grated lemon zest
- 2 (8-oz) containers lump crab meat, picked through
- 1/2 cup panko
- 1 tbsp olive oil
- 1 tbsp unsalted butter

Directions

1. Make the Creamy Sauce: Mix mayonnaise, mustards, lemon juice, hot sauce, scallion, and capers (if using).

2. Make the Crab Cakes: In a bowl, whisk together mayonnaise, egg, mustard, Worcestershire, and hot sauce. Stir in scallions, parsley, and lemon zest. Add crab and panko, mixing well. Cover and refrigerate for 1 hour.

3. Shape into eight 1-inch-thick cakes. Heat oil and butter in a skillet over medium heat and cook crab cakes in batches for 3-4 minutes per side until golden. Serve with salad and creamy sauce.

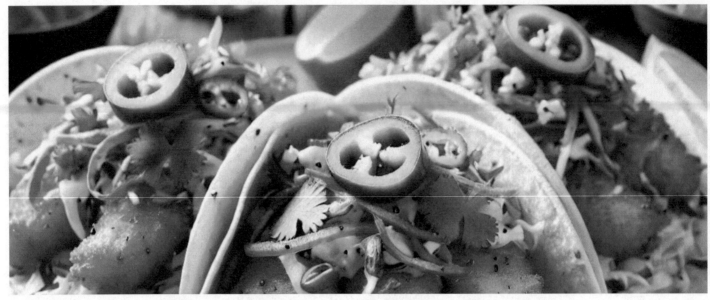

Beer-Battered Fish Tacos

Ingredients

Servings: 4

Total Time: 30 minutes

- 5 tbsp fresh lime juice (from about 2 limes), divided
- Kosher salt and pepper
- 1 small red onion, thinly sliced
- 3 tbsp sour cream
- 1/2 small green cabbage, thinly sliced
- 1 jalapeño, thinly sliced
- 1 cup all-purpose flour
- 1 tbsp cornstarch
- 1 tbsp chili powder
- 1 tsp baking powder
- 1/4 tsp cayenne
- 1 large egg, beaten
- 1 cup lager beer
- Canola oil, for frying
- 1 lb tilapia fillets, cut into strips
- 1/2 cup fresh cilantro, chopped
- 8 small flour tortillas

Directions

1.In a small bowl, mix 2 tbsp lime juice, salt, and pepper. Add onion and toss to coat. Let sit.

2.In a large bowl, whisk sour cream, remaining lime juice, salt, and pepper. Add cabbage and jalapeño, toss to coat.

3.In a bowl, whisk flour, cornstarch, chili powder, baking powder, cayenne, salt, and pepper. Add egg and beer, whisk until smooth.

4.Heat 1/2 inch oil in a skillet to 350°F. Dredge fish in dry flour mixture, then dip into beer batter. Fry until golden brown (2-3 minutes).

5.Fold cilantro into cabbage mixture. Fill tortillas with fish, slaw, and pickled onions.

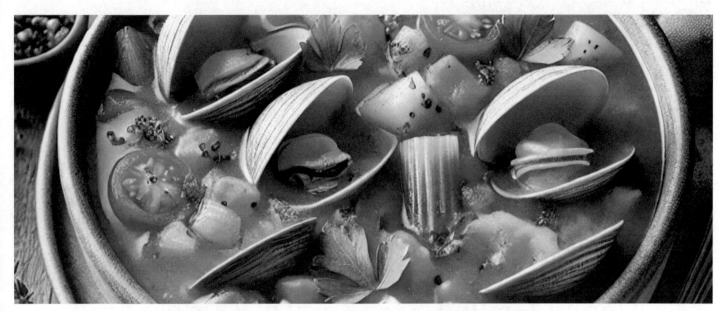

Manhattan Clam Chowder

Ingredients

Servings: 4

Total Time: 30 minutes

- 2 tbsp olive oil
- 2 stalks celery, thinly sliced
- 1 large onion, finely chopped
- 1 large carrot, cut into 1/4-inch pieces
- 2 cloves garlic, finely chopped
- 1/2 tsp red pepper flakes
- 1 lb russet potatoes, cut into 1/2-inch pieces
- 3 sprigs thyme
- 2 (8-ounce) bottles clam juice
- 1 (28-ounce) can whole tomatoes
- 1/2 cup dry white wine
- 2 (6.5-ounce) cans chopped clams, drained
- 1/4 cup flat-leaf parsley, chopped
- Crusty bread, for serving

Directions

1.Heat oil in a large pot over medium heat. Add celery, onion, and carrot, cooking for 8-10 minutes until tender. Stir in garlic and red pepper flakes, cooking for another minute.

2.Add potatoes, thyme, clam juice, tomatoes (crush them as you add), wine, and 1/2 cup water. Bring to a boil, then reduce heat and simmer for 8-10 minutes until potatoes are tender.

Stir in clams to heat through. Sprinkle with parsley and serve with crusty bread.

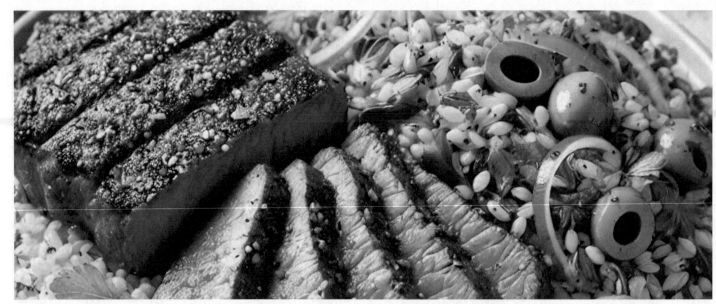

Aleppo Grilled Steak with Farro Salad

Ingredients

Servings: 4

Total Time: 25 minutes

- 1 1/2 cups quick-cooking farro
- 2 (12-oz) strip steaks, about 1 1/2 inches thick
- 3/4 tsp Aleppo pepper
- Kosher salt and pepper
- 2 tsp grated lemon zest plus 3 tbsp lemon juice
- 2 small shallots, thinly sliced
- 3 tbsp olive oil
- 3/4 cup pitted Castelvetrano olives, crushed and chopped
- 1/4 cup flat-leaf parsley, chopped
- 1/4 cup fresh mint, torn or chopped

Directions

1. Heat grill to medium. Cook farro according to package instructions.

2. Season steaks with Aleppo pepper, 1/2 tsp salt, and 1/4 tsp pepper. Grill steaks for 5-8 minutes per side for medium-rare. Let rest for at least 5 minutes before slicing.

3. In a bowl, mix lemon zest, juice, shallots, 1/2 tsp salt, and pepper, letting it sit for 5 minutes. Stir in oil and toss with farro. Fold in olives, parsley, and mint, and serve with the sliced steak.

Make-Ahead Tip: Prepare the farro salad without the herbs and refrigerate for up to two days. Add herbs just before serving.

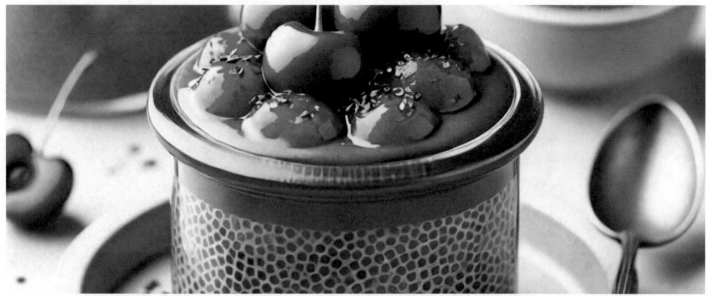

Chocolate Cherry Chia Seed Pudding

Ingredients

- Prep Time: 10 minutes
- Cook Time: 20 minutes
- Total Time: 30 minutes
- Servings: 4
- Calories: 156 kcal
- ·1 can lite coconut milk (13.5 oz)
- ·1/3 cup water
- ·2 tbsp maple syrup
- ·1/4 cup cocoa powder
- ·5 tbsp chia seeds
- ·Pinch of salt
- ·2 heaping cups frozen cherries

Directions

1.Mixing Ingredients:

 In a mixing bowl, add the coconut milk, water, maple syrup, cocoa powder, chia seeds, and a pinch of salt. Whisk them together until everything is evenly combined. Cover the bowl and place it in the fridge for at least 3 hours, or leave it overnight if you prefer.

2.Preparing Cherry Compote:

 In a saucepan, add the 2 cups of frozen cherries with 2 tablespoons of water. Cook over high heat, stirring occasionally for about 5 minutes. Then, lower the heat to medium-low and mash the cherries using a fork or potato masher. Let the mixture simmer for another 10 minutes.

3.Serving:

 Remove the cherry compote from heat and let it cool. Once ready, use both the chocolate chia seed pudding and the cherry compote to make individual servings.

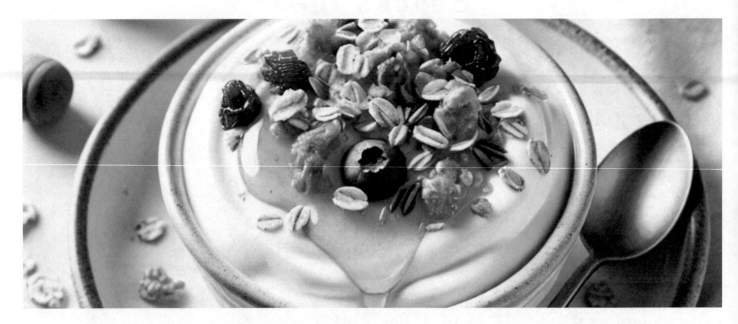

Greek Yogurt with Honey and Muesli

Ingredients

Preparation Time: 5 minutes

Makes: 1 serving

- 1/4 cup plain Greek yogurt
- 1 tsp raw honey
- 3 tbsp muesli

Directions

1.Assemble:
 Scoop the Greek yogurt into a bowl. Add 3 tablespoons of muesli and drizzle 1 teaspoon of honey on top.

2.Customize:
 You can mix and match toppings to your liking. Try adding fresh or frozen fruit, granola, nuts, coconut, or even maple syrup for a different flavor.

Tip: If you're avoiding dairy, you can substitute the yogurt with coconut, almond, or cashew yogurt.

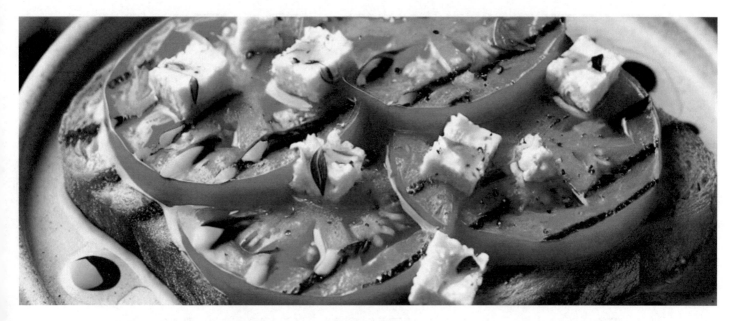

Whole Wheat Toast with Tomato

Ingredients

Preparation Time: 10 minutes

Makes: 1 serving

- 1 slice whole grain bread
- 1 tomato
- 1 tbsp extra virgin olive oil
- 2 tsp balsamic vinegar (optional)
- 1 tbsp feta cheese

Directions

1.Toast the Bread:

 Toast your slice of whole grain bread.

2.Cook Tomatoes:

 Slice the tomato and pan sear it in a non-stick pan without oil until it gets a grilled effect.

3.Assemble:

 Place the seared tomato slices on the toast. Add 1 tablespoon of feta cheese on top.

4.Finish:

 If the cheese wasn't stored in olive oil, drizzle 1 tablespoon of olive oil over the toast.

Optionally, you can drizzle balsamic vinegar on top.

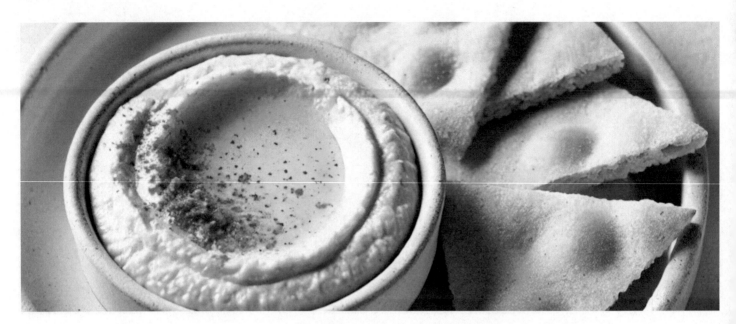

Hummus and Whole Wheat Pita

Ingredients

Preparation Time: 5 minutes

Makes: 1 serving

- 1/2-piece whole wheat pita
- 1/4 cup hummus

Directions

1.Serve:

Scoop 2 heaping tablespoons of hummus and enjoy it with toasted pita bread.

Tip: You can substitute the pita with other options like whole grain crackers, gluten-free crackers, rice crackers, or even homemade versions.

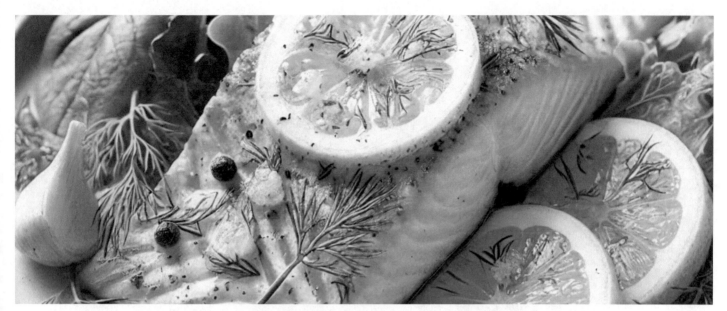

Lemon Dill Baked Salmon

Ingredients

Preparation Time: 25 minutes

Makes: 3 servings

- 425 grams salmon fillet
- 2 ¼ tsp ghee (melted)
- 1 ½ garlic cloves (minced)
- 1 ½ tbsp fresh dill (chopped)
- 3/4 lemon (zested and juiced)
- 1/8 tsp sea salt (or more to taste)
- 3 cups mixed greens

Directions

1.Preheat Oven:

 Set the oven to 375°F (191°C) and line a baking sheet with aluminum foil.

2.Prepare Salmon:

 Place the salmon fillet in the middle of the baking sheet. In a small jar, mix the melted ghee, garlic, dill, lemon juice, lemon zest, and sea salt. Pour the mixture over the salmon, then fold the foil to create a sealed pouch.

3.Bake:

 Bake the salmon for 15 to 20 minutes, or until it flakes easily with a fork.

4.Serve:

 Remove from the oven and serve the salmon with a side of mixed greens.

Tip: If you don't have ghee, you can use butter, avocado oil, or coconut oil as a substitute.

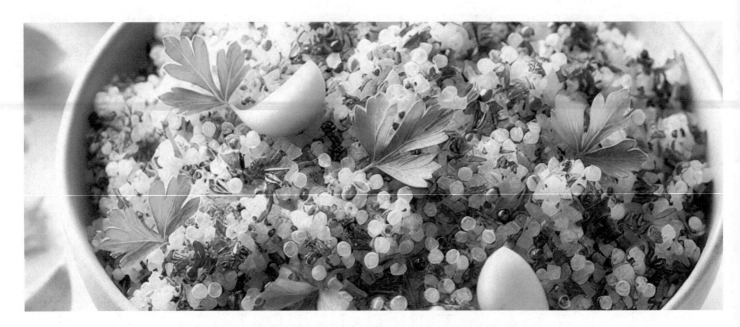

Herb and Garlic Quinoa

Ingredients

Preparation Time: 20 minutes

Makes: 5 servings

- 1 ¼ cups quinoa (dry, uncooked)
- 2 1/8 cups water
- 2 tsp extra virgin olive oil
- 1 ¼ cups parsley (finely chopped)
- 2 ½ garlic cloves (minced)
- Sea salt and black pepper (to taste)

Directions

1.Cook the Quinoa:

 Combine the quinoa and water in a pot. Bring it to a boil over high heat. Once it boils, reduce the heat to a simmer, cover the pot, and let it cook for 12 to 15 minutes or until all the water is absorbed. Remove the lid, fluff the quinoa with a fork, and set it aside.

2.Mix Ingredients:

 In a bowl, combine the cooked quinoa with olive oil, parsley, minced garlic, salt, and pepper. Mix everything well, then serve and enjoy!

Tip: You can store leftovers in an airtight container in the fridge for up to four days or freeze for up to a month. To avoid freezer burn, remove all air from the bag before freezing.

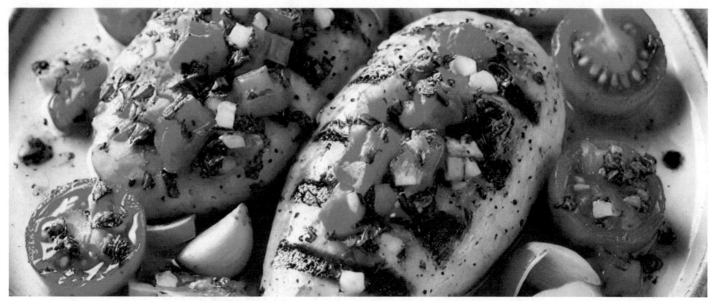

Grilled Bruschetta Chicken

Ingredients

Preparation Time: 30 minutes

Makes: 2 servings

- 227 grams chicken breast
- Sea salt and black pepper (to taste)
- 1 ½ medium tomatoes (diced)
- ¼ cup red onion (finely diced)
- 1 garlic clove (minced)
- 1 tbsp basil leaves (chopped)
- 1 ½ tsp extra virgin olive oil
- 1 ½ tsp balsamic vinegar

Directions

1.Grill the Chicken:

 Preheat your grill to medium heat. Season the chicken breasts with sea salt and black pepper. Grill for 10 to 15 minutes on each side, or until fully cooked through.

2.Prepare Bruschetta Topping:

 In a small bowl, combine diced tomatoes, red onion, garlic, chopped basil, olive oil, and balsamic vinegar. Add salt and pepper to taste.

3.Serve:

 Once the chicken is cooked, top it with the fresh bruschetta mixture.

Serving Tip: You can serve this dish with grilled or roasted vegetables, quinoa, rice, or your favorite salad. For cheese lovers, sprinkle feta, goat cheese, or shredded mozzarella on top before serving. If you don't have a grill, bake the chicken breasts in the oven at 350°F (177°C) for 30 minutes.

SHOPPING LIST

Here is a detailed and accurate shopping list based on the recipes provided, broken down into categories for ease of use. I've consolidated the ingredients for the entire set of meals (breakfast, lunch, and dinner). You can adjust quantities depending on how many servings you want to make for each meal.

Produce:

- 10 bananas
- 1 ripe banana (mashed)
- 5 cups spinach
- 2 small yellow onions
- 3 large yellow onions
- 2 small red onions
- 3 shallots
- 1/4 bulb fennel
- 3/4 cup chopped flat-leaf parsley
- 4 cups baby kale or romaine
- 1/2 cup mint leaves
- 4 stalks celery
- 2 cloves garlic
- 1 small garlic clove (minced)
- 1 garlic bulb
- 10 oz wild mushrooms
- 1 large sweet potato
- 1/2 small pineapple
- 1 pint grape tomatoes
- 1 large heirloom tomato
- 6 cherry tomatoes
- 2 medium carrots
- 1 large plum tomato
- 1 cucumber
- 1/4 ripe peach
- 1 cup cherry tomatoes
- 1/4 avocado
- 4 small potatoes
- 1 head red cabbage

- 2 medium russet potatoes
- 1 large Bartlett pear
- 1 small red chili
- 1/4 cup fresh basil (chopped)
- 1 large eggplant or 8 portobello mushrooms
- 1 small lemon
- 3/4 lemon (zested and juiced)
- 1/2 lime (juiced)
- 4 medium russet potatoes
- 5 cloves garlic (chopped)
- 1 cup fresh raspberries
- 2 cups baby arugula
- 1/2 small green cabbage
- 4 green onions
- 1 bunch green onions
- 1/4 cup scallions (chopped)
- 1/2 cup chopped walnuts
- 1/4 cup sunflower seeds
- 1/4 cup unsweetened coconut flakes
- 3 new potatoes (diced)
- 1 lime (juiced and zested)
- 1/2 cup fresh blueberries
- 1/2 cup fresh sliced strawberries
- 4 cups spinach
- 1/2 head radicchio (chopped)
- 5 cups purple cabbage
- 2-3 green onions (sliced)
- 2 medium carrots (grated)
- 2 cups sweet potato croutons
- 2 cups fresh or frozen peas
- 2 tomatoes (grilled)
- 1 avocado

Grains & Pantry:

- 6 cups old-fashioned oats
- 4 cups oat milk (or any milk of your choice)
- 1 cup steel-cut oats
- 1 cup dry quinoa
- 1 cup long-grain rice
- 1/4 cup brown sugar
- 1/2 cup maple syrup
- 1/2 cup corn syrup (or honey)
- 1/2 cup chia seeds
- 1 box (16 oz) fusilli or rotini
- 1 cup hummus
- 1 (16 oz) bottle Italian salad dressing
- 2 tbsp red wine vinegar
- 3 tbsp soy sauce
- 1 tbsp Dijon mustard
- 1/4 cup pizza sauce
- 1 jar roasted red peppers
- 4 whole-wheat tortillas
- 1 tbsp olive oil
- 1/4 cup extra virgin olive oil
- 1/4 cup coconut milk (full-fat)
- 1/4 cup panko breadcrumbs
- 1/4 cup peanut butter
- 2 tbsp tahini
- 1/4 cup unsweetened almond milk
- 2 tbsp sunflower seed butter
- 3 cups whole-wheat flour (or gluten-free)
- 1 whole-wheat English muffin
- 1 8-inch whole-wheat tortilla
- 1 loaf of whole-wheat bread
- 8 flour tortillas
- 1 can fire-roasted tomatoes
- 2 cans diced tomatoes
- 1 can black beans
- 1 can chickpeas
- 1/4 cup artichoke hearts
- 1 (13.5 oz) can light coconut milk
- 2 tbsp chopped capers
- 1 cup rolled oats
- 3 tbsp smooth almond butter
- 1/2 tsp ground ginger
- 2 tbsp balsamic vinegar
- 1/2 cup chopped almonds
- 1 package naan or flatbread
- 1 small jar plum sauce
- 1 tsp vanilla extract
- 1 tbsp toasted sesame seeds
- 1/2 tsp cumin
- 1/4 tsp smoked paprika

Dairy & Eggs:

- 6 large eggs
- 4 large eggs (separated)
- 2 cups low-fat milk (or nondairy milk)
- 12 large eggs
- 4 large eggs
- 1/2 cup grated Parmesan cheese
- 1/2 cup nonfat Greek yogurt
- 2 cups plain low-fat cottage cheese
- 6 oz shredded mozzarella
- 1/4 cup shredded sharp cheddar cheese
- 3 cups mixed shredded cheese (cheddar or Mexican blend)
- 1 container plain Greek yogurt (for snacking)
- 1 cup cheddar cheese
- 1/2 cup grated Parmesan cheese
- 1 cup shredded mozzarella cheese
- 1/4 cup feta cheese
- 1/4 cup smoked cheddar cheese
- 1/4 cup crumbled goat cheese
- 2 tbsp pepitas
- 1 cup shredded sharp cheddar cheese

Meat & Fish:

- 12 oz salmon fillets (skin on or off)
- 1 lb chicken breasts
- 1 lb lean ground pork
- 1/2 lb lean ground beef
- 1 lb shrimp (peeled and deveined)
- 1/2 lb ground turkey
- 1 lb tilapia fillets
- 1 lb sausage (andouille or other)
- 1 lb sockeye salmon (canned or fillets)
- 1 lb pork tenderloin
- 1 lb bacon (optional)
- 4 boneless skinless chicken thighs

Canned & Jarred Goods:

- 2 tbsp mustard (whole-grain, Dijon)
- 1 jar peanut butter
- 1 small jar of pickles
- 2 cans black beans
- 1 jar salsa
- 1 can low-sodium chicken broth
- 2 (8-oz) cans clams (chopped)

Spices & Seasonings:

- Ground black pepper
- Kosher salt
- 1 tsp cumin
- 1/4 tsp ground cinnamon
- 1/2 tsp ground nutmeg
- 1 tsp paprika
- 1/4 tsp cayenne pepper
- 1/2 tsp smoked paprika
- 1 tsp Italian seasoning
- 1 tsp garlic powder
- 1 tsp red pepper flakes
- 2 tsp baking soda

This list covers most ingredients you'll need to make all the recipes for breakfasts, lunches, and dinners.

30-DAYS MEAL PLAN

Week 1

Day 1
- Breakfast: Basic Banana Overnight Oats
- Lunch: Healthy Italian Pasta Salad
- Dinner: Miso Glazed Salmon with Snap Peas

Day 2
- Breakfast: Easy Broccoli and Cheese Egg Bake
- Lunch: Crockpot Lentil Soup
- Dinner: Cajun Shrimp and Sausage Skillet

Day 3
- Breakfast: Sheet Pan Breakfast Sandwiches
- Lunch: Fully-Loaded Veggie Sandwiches
- Dinner: Red Lentil Dal

Day 4
- Breakfast: The Ultimate High Protein Scrambled Eggs
- Lunch: Salmon Salad Tartines
- Dinner: Healthy Pork Lettuce Wraps

Day 5
- Breakfast: Berry and Chia Overnight Oats
- Lunch: Simple Pasta Salad
- Dinner: Quinoa and Shrimp Grits

Day 6
- Breakfast: Light and Fluffy Cottage Cheese Pancakes
- Lunch: Salmon BLT Salad with Chive Ranch Dressing
- Dinner: Sesame Peanut Noodles

Day 7
- Breakfast: Make-Ahead Veggie Breakfast Burrito
- Lunch: Waldorf Chicken Salad
- Dinner: Baked Chicken Cutlets with Pineapple Rice

Week 2
Day 8
- Breakfast: Winter Citrus Yogurt Bowl
- Lunch: Snap Pea and Chicken Salad
- Dinner: Baked Tilapia with Radish Relish

Day 9
- Breakfast: Strawberry Cream Smoothie
- Lunch: Poblano and Black Bean Loaded Baked Potato
- Dinner: Slow Cooker Chicken Marbella

Day 10
- Breakfast: Egg and Avocado Toast
- Lunch: Vegetarian Antipasto Salad
- Dinner: Sesame Chicken with Chili Lime Slaw

Day 11
- Breakfast: Almond Butter Oatmeal
- Lunch: Fiery Black Bean Soup
- Dinner: Quick and Easy Taco Salad

Day 12
- Breakfast: Make-Ahead Egg Casserole
- Lunch: Salmon Niçoise Salad
- Dinner: Mediterranean Baked Cod

Day 13
- Breakfast: Sweet Potato Breakfast Hash
- Lunch: Air Fryer Salmon Flatbreads
- Dinner: Grilled Bruschetta Chicken

Day 14
- Breakfast: Apple Crumble Muffins
- Lunch: Salmon BLT Salad with Chive Ranch Dressing
- Dinner: Aleppo Grilled Steak with Farro Salad

Day 15
- Breakfast: Blueberry AIP-Paleo Breakfast Bars
- Lunch: Salmon Niçoise Salad
- Dinner: Sheet Pan Chickpea Chicken

Day 16
- Breakfast: Spinach & Egg Scramble with Raspberries
- Lunch: Healthy Tuna Salad with Cranberries
- Dinner: Wild Mushroom Frittata with Cheddar, Green Onions, and Peas

Day 17
- Breakfast: Sriracha, Egg & Avocado Overnight Oats
- Lunch: Salmon Salad Tartines
- Dinner: Sweet Potato Cheddar BBQ Chicken Burgers

Day 18
- Breakfast: Peanut Energy Bars
- Lunch: Snap Pea and Chicken Salad
- Dinner: Garlicky Shrimp and White Bean Toast

Day 19
- Breakfast: Raspberry-Peach-Mango Smoothie Bowl
- Lunch: Fully-Loaded Veggie Sandwiches
- Dinner: Spring Green Detox Soup

Day 20
- Breakfast: Avocado & Kale Omelet
- Lunch: Healthy Italian Pasta Salad
- Dinner: Crab Cakes and Creamy Sauce

Day 21
- Breakfast: Cocoa-Chia Pudding with Raspberries
- Lunch: Salmon Salad Tartines
- Dinner: Manhattan Clam Chowder

Week 4

Day 22
- Breakfast: Muffin-Tin Quiches with Smoked Cheddar & Potato
- Lunch: Simple Pasta Salad
- Dinner: 30-Minute Thai Chicken Curry

Day 23
- Breakfast: Spinach & Egg Sweet Potato Toast
- Lunch: Poblano and Black Bean Loaded Baked Potato
- Dinner: Pear and Prosciutto Pizza

Day 24
- Breakfast: Baked Oatmeal with Pears
- Lunch: Waldorf Chicken Salad
- Dinner: Steak and Cauliflower Potatoes with Sautéed Spinach

Day 25
- Breakfast: Southwestern Waffle
- Lunch: Salmon Niçoise Salad
- Dinner: Oven-Roasted Salmon with Charred Lemon Vinaigrette

Day 26
- Breakfast: Savory Oatmeal with Cheddar, Collards & Eggs
- Lunch: Snap Pea and Chicken Salad
- Dinner: Baked Tilapia with Radish Relish

Day 27
- Breakfast: Peanut Butter & Chia Berry Jam English Muffin
- Lunch: Fiery Black Bean Soup
- Dinner: Sesame Chicken with Chili Lime Slaw

Day 28
- Breakfast: Parmesan Cloud Eggs
- Lunch: Salmon Salad Tartines

Dinner: Beer-Battered Fish Tacos

Week 5 (Days 29-30)

Day 29

- **Breakfast: Red Berry Smoothies**
- **Lunch: Salmon Salad Tartines**
- **Dinner: Herb and Garlic Quinoa with Lemon Dill Baked Salmon**

Day 30

- **Breakfast: Peanut Butter-Banana Roll-Ups**
- **Lunch: Air Fryer Salmon Flatbreads**
- **Dinner: Grilled Bruschetta Chicken**

Scan to Get
Dr Barbara Inspired 15 Day Liver
Cleanse
for Free

Made in the USA
Columbia, SC
29 December 2024

50828410R00063